The Menopause

ask the experts

The Menopause

ask the experts

Compiled and edited by
Norma Goldman

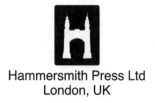

Hammersmith Press Ltd
London, UK

First published in 2009 by Hammersmith Press Limited
496 Fulham Palace Road, London SW6 6JD, UK
www.hammersmithpress.co.uk

Disclaimer

While every care has been taken, the editor accepts no responsibility for damage or illness that results from advice or information given in this book.

If you are worried about any symptoms you are experiencing or you have medical problems, always consult a health professional first. Every woman is unique and what suits one woman may not suit another. Therefore, the information and advice in this book should not take the place of advice from your GP, gynaecologist or any other qualified health professional.

Studies quoted and information included in this book were correct at the time of going to press and may be out of date by the time this book is read.

British Library Cataloguing in Publication Data: a CIP record of this book is available from the British Library.

ISBN 978-1-905140-24-4

Designed by Julie Bennett
Production by Helen Whitehorn, Pathmedia
Printed and bound by TJ International Ltd, UK
Cover image: © Joe McDonald/CORBIS

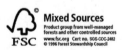

Mixed Sources
Product group from well-managed forests and other controlled sources
www.fsc.org Cert no. SGS-COC-2482
© 1996 Forest Stewardship Council
FSC

Contents

Acknowledgements   vii

The Experts   viii

Introduction – A few chance words along the way   xii

1. General information   1

2. Symptoms   9
     General symptoms   10
     Hot flushes and night sweats   13
     Joint problems and arthritis   16
     Bladder and vaginal changes   18
     Skin, hair and mouth problems   22
     Emotional symptoms   28
     Weight and digestive problems   34

3. Osteoporosis   37

4. HRT (Hormone Replacement Therapy)   43

5. Complementary therapies   70

Contents

6. Nutrition   **78**
    General nutrition   79
    Phytoestrogens   85
    Vitamins and minerals   89

7. A mixture of options for coping with the menopause   **101**

8. Women's health and general health issues   **120**
    Breast cancer   120
    Hysterectomy   123
    Fibroids   124
    Endometriosis   126
    Miscellaneous problems   127

Appendix: HRT and breast cancer risk   **135**

Glossary   **139**

References   **145**

Contact details of organisations   **148**

Index   **152**

Acknowledgements

Thanks go to the members of The Menopause Exchange, especially to those of you who have provided the questions for this book and shared your experiences with us. Without these, this book could not have come about.

I should like to thank my panel of experts for their expertise in answering the questions sent in on a wide variety of topics by members of The Menopause Exchange.

I am grateful to Georgina Bentliff at Hammersmith Press for publishing **The Menopause: ask the experts** and enabling my idea to come to fruition.

I should like to thank my daughter Victoria Goldman, who is a health journalist, for her invaluable help and advice as I compiled the book.

I should like to thank my daughter Rebecca Levene for her encouragement and interest.

Thanks go to my PA, Nicola Duckworth, for her assistance.

Finally, a big thank you to my husband, Alan, for allowing the word 'menopause' to become a household word and for his support and encouragement.

The Experts

Kathy Abernethy RN

Kathy Abernethy is associate director/senior nurse specialist at the Menopause Clinical and Research Unit, North West London Hospitals NHS Trust, Northwick Park Hospital, Harrow, Middlesex. She is director of 'the menopause course' – an educational initiative for nurses. Kathy is chair of the Royal College of Nursing National Menopause Group and a member of the educational sub-committee of the British Menopause Society.

Gaynor Bussell BSc (Hons) RD RPHNutr. MIFST

Gaynor Bussell is a nutrition scientist and dietitian and works as nutrition manager for the Food and Drink Federation. Her freelance work includes running a private patients' dietetic clinic and advising a number of women's health organisations. She has specialised in women's health for 16 years. Her other specialist areas are public health and vitamins and minerals.

Dr Kathryn Clement MRCOG

Dr Kathryn Clement is a specialist registrar in obstetrics and gynaecology with a special interest in menopausal health and contraception. She is working at Graingerville Clinic, Newcastle-upon-Tyne with Dr Diana Mansour.

Mr Michael Dooley MMs MFFP FRCOG

Mr Michael Dooley is a consultant in obstetrics and gynaecology at Dorset County Hospital in Dorchester. He also consults at The Lister Hospital and in Harley Street, London. His special interests include the menopause, osteoporosis, premenstrual syndrome, period problems, endometriosis and polycystic ovarian syndrome.

Dr Sarah Gray BSc (Hons) MBBS MRCGP DRCOG DFFP FHEA

Dr Sarah Gray is a GP who specialises in all aspects of women's health. She is a council member of the British Menopause Society and runs the Specialist Menopause Service in Cornwall. She is extensively involved in teaching and training healthcare professionals as well as educating women directly so that as many as possible have the chance to make informed decisions about their own health.

Dr Sally Hope MA (Oxon) FRCGP DRCOG

Dr Sally Hope is a GP in Woodstock, Oxfordshire. She is deputy editor of *Menopause International* and the RCGP representative for osteoporosis on the NICE clinical guidelines committee.

Angie Jefferson RD RPHNutr

Angie Jefferson is a consultant dietitian, who has run her own consultancy practice for the past 10 years. Whether communicating face to face, via the web or in written form, Angie focuses on delivering simple positive messages for achieving optimum nutrition within a healthy lifestyle. In addition to the practical application of the science of nutrition, Angie's specialties include women's and children's nutrition, functional foods, weight management and heart health.

Dr Nicola Mullin MRCOG, MFFP

Dr Nicola Mullin is a consultant in sexual and reproductive health, Western Cheshire Primary Care Trust. She is chair of the education committee of the Faculty of Sexual and Reproductive Health and chair of the North West Society for Family Planning and Sexual Medicine. Her special interests are the menopause, contraception at the perimenopause, management of symptoms for younger women with breast cancer and the development of community gynaecology services.

Dani Singer MBACP / UKCP

Dani Singer is a specialist counsellor and psychotherapist at the Menopause Clinical & Research Unit, North West London Hospitals NHS Trust, Northwick Park Hospital, Harrow, Middlesex, and at the PMS Clinic, Queen Charlotte's & Chelsea Hospital, London. Her special interests are the psychological aspects of menopause transition and premature menopause. She has co-edited and contributed to books on the menopause.

Dr Nuttan K Tanna MRPharmS, DComP, PhD

Dr Nuttan Tanna is a consultant pharmacist in women's healthcare and older people, menopause and osteoporosis. She is associate director of pharmacy practice, research and development at the Menopause Clinical & Research Unit, North West London Hospitals NHS Trust, Northwick Park Hospital, Harrow, Middlesex and is co-chair of the North West London Osteoporosis & Fracture Forum. Her special interest topics are menopause, osteoporosis, falls and fractures.

Lila Thakerar MRPharmS

Lila Thakerar is a community pharmacist, having won two national business awards in 2005. She writes for magazines and national newspapers and advises and writes about the menopause, smoking and NHS services to the community. She is also a spokesperson for the National Pharmacy Association.

All are or have been members of the experts panel of:

The Menopause Exchange,
PO Box 205, Bushey, Herts WD23 1ZS
Tel: 020 8420 7245
Fax: 020 8954 2783
Email: norma@menopause-exchange.co.uk
Web: www.menopause-exchange.co.uk

Introduction

A few chance words along the way

I have called this introduction 'A few chance words along the way' because it really was a fortunate series of events that led me to where I am today, a case of being in the right place at the right time. When I qualified as a pharmacist in 1966, I never expected to have a change in career 32 years later. Fortunately, I was brave enough to grab opportunities whenever they arose. One thing led to another – and, as they say, the rest is history.

In 1992, I was invited to attend a short health promotion course in my capacity as pharmacist. I was so fascinated by the concept of promoting good health, rather than just treating ill-health, that I enrolled on a three-year Master's degree course in health promotion the following year. I qualified as a health promotion specialist in 1996.

During my Master's degree, I wrote an assessment of a menopause course for a fictitious women's group and a dissertation on health promotion for women at midlife and the menopause. I don't know what prompted me to choose this topic. I obtained my Master's degree when I was 52, about the age of the menopause. However, I wasn't experiencing menopausal symptoms myself, so I didn't need any personal answers.

In 1997, at a family gathering, I bumped into an old acquaintance. We had studied pharmacy together many years before. When he asked me about my career, I said that I was thinking of changing direction and that I was currently interested in the menopause. A week later, he contacted me with a fantastic opportunity. Would I present a talk on the menopause for women in a pharmacy? Not surprisingly, I jumped at the chance. Thanks to my time researching the menopause, the presentation was a success. It was just the first of many presentations to both women and health professionals in a variety of settings, including organisations, charities, women's groups, workplaces and exhibitions. Over ten years later, my presentations are still going strong.

Whilst carrying out research for my presentations, one of the librarians I met mentioned that she had seen a menopause newsletter in a library abroad. Since she was going through the menopause, she wished that someone would write a newsletter in the UK. I had already identified a lack of unbiased information on the subject, so this gave me an idea. With the help of my daughter, who is a health journalist, I founded The Menopause Exchange in 1999 to launch *The Menopause Exchange Newsletter*. Our aim was to provide unbiased and practical information on all aspects of the menopause and issues around midlife. In summer 2000, we expanded our services with an 'Ask the Experts' panel. This was then followed by quarterly fact sheets and an information service.

The 'Ask the Experts' panel now consists of 11 members, all of whom have professional expertise in the menopause and long experience of answering the real-life questions of women with menopausal symptoms. The panel includes menopause consultants, GPs, a specialist menopause nurse, a specialist menopause pharmacist, a community pharmacist, two dietitians and a counsellor. Because our members send in the questions, we're not responsible for the subject matter or content; it's interesting to see what women worry about the most.

Many of our members have told us that the 'Ask the Experts' panel's answers have helped them through their menopause. By putting some of the questions and answers into book form, I hope that this will help other women with similar concerns. It's natural to be interested in other women's experiences and it can help to know that there are other women in 'the same boat'. However, every woman is unique and what suits one will not suit another. So you must look at your own situation before using any advice given in this book and discuss it with a health professional.

This book is for women who are approaching or at the menopause, younger women who have had a premature menopause or hysterectomy, and post-menopausal women. It is also aimed at health professionals working in this field. Remember that no menopausal woman needs to suffer unnecessarily and it's important that you obtain help for distressing symptoms.

Norma Goldman
2009

Chapter 1

General information

All women go through the menopause. The menopause means your 'last menstrual period', but the term is now widely used to describe the 'change of life' that occurs around this time. The menopause is recognised to have occurred after 12 consecutive months of no periods.

As you approach the menopause, your ovaries produce less and less of the female hormones oestrogen and progesterone and you produce eggs less regularly. In most women, these changes don't take place overnight and they can last for several years. During this time, your monthly periods may become irregular, occur only occasionally, become more frequent or become heavier and last longer. You may also notice some spotting between them. Eventually, your ovaries will stop producing hormones and your egg production and monthly periods will finally stop completely.

For most women, changes in their periods begin in their late 40s, with their last period occurring at an average age of 51. It's a very individual experience. Some women don't experience symptoms at all, while others have a dreadful time.

The menopause is not all doom and gloom, however, and some women find that there is a positive side. No more monthly periods is just one benefit. The menopause can be a time to discover new opportunities, using your experiences and reflection, and it is often an important milestone. Women can live as much as one third of their life after the menopause, so there's plenty of time to take on new ideas and challenges. I am an example of a woman who changed direction at the menopause, and I hope that this encourages other women to 'have a go'.

***

I am confused about the different stages of the menopause. Please can you tell me what they are and what can happen at each stage?

The early stage of the menopause is described as the perimenopause. This may start some months or occasionally years before your periods actually stop. It is the time when hormonal fluctuations commonly occur and you may start to see menopausal-type symptoms (see page 9), such as flushes and sweats. This may be when you begin to see a change in the pattern of your periods, perhaps getting less regular and maybe even missing some months altogether. This leads into the menopause itself, which is simply the occurrence of the last menstrual bleed. Around the time of the last period, many women experience menopausal symptoms and these can be troublesome. Once you have not seen a period for 12 months, you are described as post-menopausal and usually your symptoms lessen, although they can continue for anything from a few weeks to a few years.

What influences our experience of the menopause?

It is possible that our expectations of the menopause may in-fluence how we experience it. For example, if our mother or sister had a bad time, then we may expect to do so as well, even though this is not necessarily the case. Previous depression, particularly forms relating to hormones, such as premenstrual syndrome and post-natal depression, may lead to feelings of depression during the menopause. Cultural beliefs may affect your experience too – for example, is the menopause seen as a time of failure or the beginning of old age? Or, are older women respected and valued in your culture? Such factors may influence how you actually feel about the menopause and how you respond to some of the symptoms. However, the most common symptom, hot flushes, happens to all sorts of women in the UK of many different cultures, even to the most positive thinking! The other main factor influencing how you experience the menopause is in the suddenness of its onset – a surgical menopause, for example, is likely to cause more symp-toms than a natural one.

I had a hysterectomy recently at the age of 37. I still have my ovaries. At what age should I expect to go through the menopause?

Your ovaries were conserved at the time of your hysterectomy, so they should continue to function normally. However, in some women who still have their ovaries after a hysterectomy the menopause will be brought forward by about two years (the average age of the menopause is 51). Occasionally, ovaries stop working much sooner than this, perhaps partly due to a change in the blood supply to the uterus. As you won't have outward signs of when the menopause occurs (that is, changes associated with periods), you will need to rely on the presence of symptoms (see page 9) to tell when the menopause has happened. A simple blood test can help confirm this, although blood tests may be misleading in some cases.

I am 57 and have not yet had any signs of the menopause. Is this unusual?

Unusual yes, but not abnormal! Although the average age of the menopause is usually described as 51, there is wide variation. Some women may, quite naturally, experience menopause in their late 40s. Others, like you, will see periods until 57 or 58. It is likely that your periods will stop soon, but that does not mean you will necessarily feel worse for it. You may escape symptoms like hot flushes.

My menopause and overactive thyroid seemed to come together – is there any connection?

Generally these are entirely separate problems that have happened to coincide. It is, however, possible that both are due, at least in part, to an autoimmune reaction. An autoimmune reaction is a type of response where your body produces antibodies to tissues of your own body. These antibodies generally have an inactivating effect, but they can sometimes stimulate the thyroid gland, making it appear to be overactive. Blood tests can detect whether thyroid-stimulating antibodies are present. These tests are routinely performed to advise on the most appropriate treatment. If you decide to take hormone replacement therapy (HRT), this can affect thyroid hormone levels and your doctor should be aware of the potential for interaction.

What is an early menopause and what causes it?

The average age of the menopause is 51 years with the usual age range being between 45 and 55 years. If the menopause occurs before the age of 45 years, it is said to be 'early' and if it occurs before the age of 40 it is said to be 'premature'. Some women undergo an early or premature menopause due to treatments for cancer; removal of the ovaries by surgery causes an immediate menopause. For most women however, there is no obvious reason why their periods stopped prematurely. There is thought to be a genetic link, so if your mother underwent an early menopause there is a chance that you may too. A woman undergoing a premature menopause should take HRT until around the age of 50 so that she can continue to have oestrogen for the same amount of time as her peer group, whose ovaries still work normally.

(Editor's note: Some gynaecologists consider menopause before the age of 45 years to be premature.)

I didn't go through the menopause until I was 52. However, my 35-year-old daughter has just been told that she is going through a premature menopause. Her 30-year-old sister is now concerned that she could experience the menopause early as well. Do you have any advice for my daughters?

The incidence of premature menopause in the UK is about 1 per cent in women under 40 years. There can be a familial tendency between sisters, but although you are right to be concerned about your younger daughter, there is little that can prevent the onset of menopause. She may want to investigate her future fertility options, including having some diagnostic tests that could help to predict the likelihood of imminent menopause; for example, blood tests measure oestrogen levels which indicate the activity of the ovaries and can help to identify if the menopause might happen soon. However, these tests are only an indication. They also may not be available on the NHS. Cyopreservation (freezing) of ovarian tissue is becoming more readily available, although it is usually reserved for women with a diagnosis of cancer. A gynaecologist would be the person to discuss this with.

Your older daughter may be struggling to come to terms with a number of issues in her life. The experience of menopause at a young age can be very isolating, and the symptoms can be bad enough at any time without a loss of natural fertility at a young age as well. The charity Daisy Network, Premature Menopause Support Group can provide information and support. A special referral to a menopause clinic is recommended in the interests of her physical and emotional wellbeing.

What are menopause clinics, how do I obtain an appointment and what does a consultation involve?

Most women with menopausal symptoms can be seen and successfully treated by their GP or practice nurse, but sometimes referral to a specialist menopause clinic may be necessary – for example, if you have tried various therapies with little success, have had medical illnesses that make treatments hard to find or if you need specialist advice, perhaps because of an early menopause or previous breast cancer. Such clinics will take a detailed medical history and make a full assessment before deciding on a course of action for you as an individual. Sometimes, they can offer treatments not available to GPs. Other team members (e.g. a counsellor, pharmacist or dietitian) may also see you; these professionals work together to provide a service that is more specialised than most GPs can offer. Such clinics may refer directly to other services such as bone density measurement or breast clinic services. To get an appointment, you will need to be referred by your GP.

I'm worried about my mother, who I think is going through the menopause. I'm sure she's having hot flushes. We're an Asian family and my mother doesn't like to talk about the menopause. Is there anything special about the way in which Asians experience the menopause?

All women go through the menopause, as this is a natural end to a woman's reproductive phase or ability to have children. The average age for the menopause is around 51, but it can occur any time between the ages of 45 and 55. Typical symptoms include hot flushes, night sweats and patterns of irregular erratic bleeding. Some work suggests that Asian women may go through the menopause a few years earlier then Caucasian women.

Generally, Asian women don't openly talk about sensitive matters, including the menopause, with male and younger members of the family. It may also be that they are not aware of what going through the menopause actually means. Some women may think that their feeling unwell due to hot flushes and night sweats means accepting that they can't care for their family as well as they should do, so they may not raise or talk about this issue. Research on Asian cultural values[1, 2] suggests that older Asian women actually welcome 'old age' as they stop having monthly bleeds, and therefore feel freer when it comes to carrying out daily religious activities. It has been noted that within joint Asian family systems, older women members are regarded as wiser and more experienced and their advice is often sought by younger family members. This role earns them respect from their family, which they like.

With regards to your mother, there are leaflets available on the menopause in various Asian languages in the UK. You could get these from your local hospital menopause service for her to read through. If she requires further information on the menopause, she can discuss this with her GP (with you accompanying her for support if she wants) or ask for a referral to the local hospital menopause service. If she is aware of the menopause but is unwilling to consider treatment in the form of hormone replacement therapy (she may have heard that this has various side effects and risks), then she would benefit from discussing this with her GP or hospital menopause service. If she has good-quality information provided within a supportive environment, she may feel more able to ask questions openly, raise her concerns and accept ongoing treatment that she is comfortable with.

(Editor's note: Joint families are important for Asian families, as it is expected that parents will be looked after by their son and daughter-in-law and live with them, so that their old age is comfortable.)

Chapter 2
Symptoms

Your menopausal symptoms may begin to appear when your ovaries start to 'wind down' and then gradually stop producing the hormone oestrogen. The most common are hot flushes and night sweats, which affect around 75 per cent of women.

This chapter includes sections on general or non-specific menopausal symptoms, hot flushes and night sweats, joint problems and arthritis, bladder and vaginal changes, skin, hair and mouth problems, emotional symptoms and weight and digestive problems. Although the list of possible symptoms is virtually endless, bear in mind that some women don't experience any and that many women experience one or two only. The type, severity and duration vary from woman to woman.

The menopause comes at a time of life when you may be experiencing physical, emotional and social changes that can affect how you experience certain menopausal symptoms. You should also bear in mind that some medical conditions or medications can cause some of the symptoms mentioned, which is why it is important to seek medical advice.

Some women speak to their friends and family about their symptoms, but others are more reticent or too embarrassed to do this. They may not even be comfortable about consulting their doctor or a health professional, especially if they are experiencing any bladder, vaginal and emotional problems. Hopefully this chapter will highlight the fact that help is available and that you shouldn't be embarrassed to ask for it.

***

General symptoms

I am approaching the menopause. What are the most common menopausal symptoms and at what stage of the menopause can they occur?

The menopause (last period) usually occurs around the age of 51, but it's not uncommon to get symptoms in the couple of years leading up to it, as well as after periods have actually stopped. In fact, symptoms can be worse in the times of hormonal fluctuation leading up to the last actual period. About 75 per cent of women experience hot flushes or night sweats, some only mildly, others more intensely. These are the commonest symptoms. Quite a few women describe symptoms such as poor concentration, memory loss and mood swings too, again often before periods stop for good. Some women have no symptoms at all and for most women they are gone completely within a year to 18 months. Only a minority continue to have symptoms for a long time after their last period.

I am 44. I am going through the perimenopause and I haven't had a period for three months. I have my ovaries

and womb. I am not taking HRT or any other medication. Since I have been going through the menopause, I have been suffering from giddiness coinciding with anxiety. Things that never annoyed me before are becoming big issues. I have suffered from vertigo in the past but it went away. Please can you give me some advice.

There are a number of issues here. Are you sure you are perimenopausal and not pregnant? In a 44 year old who is dizzy and hasn't had a period for three months, I'd always check. Also if you really are perimenopausal, you should seriously consider HRT, as menopause under 45 is considered 'premature'. Dizziness may be vertigo (a disabling sensation in which the affected individual feels that either he himself or his surroundings are in a state of constant movement), in which case you should be referred to an ear, nose and throat clinic (ENT clinic), and there are medications like betahistine that your GP can prescribe. Your blood pressure should also be checked (too high or very low can both make you dizzy), and a haemoglobin blood test carried out to exclude anaemia.

I am an aromatherapist. Quite a few of my patients in the menopause age group complain of headaches. Is this a menopause symptom and if so, why does it occur at the menopause?

All sorts of headaches (tension and true migraines) are worse around the time of a menstrual period, and get better after the period. This may be due to various hormones (such as progestogen) or neurotransmitters. At the perimenopause (the two to three years before periods stop), all the hormones are in chaos, so it's not surprising that headaches get worse. The great news is that after all periods stop forever, headaches including migraine get less frequent. The other practical point to mention is that around the age of 50, your eyes change rapidly and some women need glasses for the first time. They may get headaches from trying to squint at a computer screen with the wrong specs.

I am 46 and have irregular periods. I have been sterilised. I am taking thyroxine tablets – 25 micrograms daily – because I had a sub-total thyroidectomy due to Grave's disease. I have osteoporosis. I suffer with hot flushes and palpitations. How can I cope with the palpitations which can occur about three or four times a day? Does HRT help palpitations?

Palpitations can occur for a variety of reasons, but can be part of the range of symptoms experienced at menopause. Your irregular periods suggest that the process of menopause transition is already under way. An overactive thyroid can be responsible, but this won't be the case if you are being monitored by your GP. You need further investigation if the palpitations make you feel unwell, light-headed or breathless. The first thing to do is to ask your GP to check your heart rhythm with an ECG. If this is normal, I would first suggest cutting out stimulants such as caffeine. If this does not solve your problem, you may consider hormone replacement therapy (HRT). On the basis of the information given, this could potentially relieve both your flushes and palpitations and provide protection for your bones.

I am 56 and two years post-menopausal. I experience palpitations, which started four years ago but have been worse in the last year. My heart checks have been normal, but I now take beta-blockers. I have tried to reduce the dose, to no avail. I have put on weight since taking them and they have slowed me down. What causes palpitations if heart tests are normal? Can they be a menopausal symptom?

Palpitations are a classic symptom of the menopause, although the mechanism causing them is not understood. They can be made worse by caffeine (cut out tea, coffee and fizzy drinks), alcohol, tiredness and stress. A lot of people get fast heart beats, sometimes called supraventricular tachycardias (SVTs). SVTs are a nuisance and can be frightening, but they don't shorten your life. If you have been checked out, that is great. SVTs can be treated with various drugs (e.g. beta-blockers or verapamil) if you get symptoms. The trick is to be on the lowest possible dose, so you get the least side effects, or to change the drug or just accept the side effects. I have patients on half a tablet of the lowest dose beta-blocker; you can try cutting down, or ask your GP to change you to a different medication. The major 'side effect' of beta-blockers is that you live longer!

Hot flushes and night sweats

When I have a hot flush I get tingling down my arms and an unpleasant 'pressure' sensation in my head. What causes this?

A hot flush occurs when your body attempts to lose heat by diverting blood to the blood vessels in the skin of your upper body. Tingling down your arms may be caused by the sudden influx of blood into your skin. Alternatively, some people breathe much faster when they are having a hot flush and this 'hyperventilation' can cause tingling in the arms and fingers and around the mouth. Any symptoms related to hyperventilation can be prevented or stopped by calm slow breathing. Some people find breathing into a paper bag helpful. The unpleasant pressure sensation in your head may be explained by a dramatic increase in blood flow to your face and scalp. Unfortunately, there is limited information available to explain your symptoms, although these are very common in menopausal women.

Last summer, I felt hot and sweaty on a number of occasions. I am 48 and have not experienced any signs of the menopause. I don't know if this will recur this summer. How will I know whether I am experiencing hot flushes or whether it is simply a reaction to the good weather?

Although the menopause commonly occurs around the age of 51, it's not unusual for some symptoms, such as hot flushes, to start earlier, even before the periods stop. So it may be that you are experiencing the early stages of the perimenopause (the stage before actual menopause), leading to occasional flushes which are worsened by the hot weather. You can't really know for sure until your period pattern changes, but the advice is the same, whatever the cause. Wear light layers of clothing, drink plenty of fluids (non alcoholic!) and avoid situations that might make your flushes worse, such as stressful environments or sudden changes in temperature. Other things that worsen flushes include caffeine, alcohol and spicy foods, so keep this in mind during the summer months.

Is there any connection between what happens during a hot flush and an increase in the heart rate/or an irregular heart beat?

Hot flushes are episodes of inappropriate heat loss by the body. The heat loss is achieved by widespread opening up of superficial blood vessels in your upper body. A hot flush will increase your heart rate, but shouldn't cause an irregular beat.

Normally, the blood vessels in your skin are constricted to maintain your body heat. When they are opened up to allow blood flow through them, the heart has to pump faster to get the same volume of blood through a larger network of pipes. Unfortunately, our understanding of flushes is still unclear and requires further research.

Every woman experiences oestrogen loss at the time of the menopause. So why do some women have such awful hot flushes and others experience none? It is two and a half years since my last period and my flushes are as bad as ever! How much longer do you think they will keep going and why hasn't my body adjusted by now to the oestrogen loss?

Hot flushes and night sweats are two of the most common symptoms associated with the menopause, affecting around three in four women. The flushes often start before the periods stop and are most frequent in the first year after the final menstrual period. Although the flushes are usually present for less than five years, a few women will continue to flush beyond the age of 60.

A woman's perception and experience of the menopause are influenced by biological factors (e.g. general health, weight), and emotional and social factors (e.g. expectations of what the menopause will be like). Keeping fit and active, avoiding smoking and trying to be positive about this stage of your life will all help; but ultimately the rate of fall and fluctuations in your oestrogen levels and the time it takes to adjust are very individual.

I'm sorry that you are having such trouble with your flushes; why not discuss with your doctor a short trial of low-dose HRT?

My hot flushes seem to be getting worse, especially during the day while I am at work. How can I speak to my work colleagues about this without feeling embarrassed?

Understanding colleagues will make your life easier, so it is a good idea to mention the hot flushes to them. Wear layers of clothing made from natural fibres, have a glass of cold water to sip and a fan on your desk. You could move your desk closer to a window or away from a radiator. Try to learn to breathe slowly and keep relaxed during a flush; making light of what's happening is often better than getting stressed and upset.

Joint problems and arthritis

My joints feel a little stiff when I get up in the morning. Could this be a symptom of the menopause? Do you have any tips?

One of the most striking things about the menopause is the joint stiffness. One of the immediate effects of HRT is that you stop feeling stiff. Women find coming off HRT that they noticeably stiffen up. Like most symptoms of the menopause, the stiffness gets better over about a year. A good treatment is glucosamine, which is a natural non-toxic compound that has been shown to help repair and maintain cartilage. Moderate exercise, like a brisk 20-minute walk every day, will keep your heart and circulation fit and help stop your bones thinning too.

Are you consuming enough calcium and vitamin D in your diet? Most women don't have enough calcium, and can either drink more milk or take a calcium supplement. There are, of course, some rare diseases like polymyalgia rheumatica, or some of the inflammatory arthritides that can start with severe muscle aching or early morning stiffness, so if you are really suffering, see your GP for a check-up.

I am 52. I suffered the onset of osteoarthritis (specifically cervical spondylosis, which is a spinal condition resulting from degeneration and flattening of the intervertebral discs in the cervical (neck) region) about four years ago. I have physiotherapy during bad flare-ups and take glucosamine and cod liver oil. I try to eat well, rest and do gentle exercise. During the last year my periods have almost finished and hot flushes arrived. I started taking soya tablets and soya milk. The flushes completely disappeared for several months but then returned. I experience hot flushes every two-three hours day and night. My arthritis flares up if I get cold so I wrap up and when I am indoors I sweat and become

exhausted. I was advised by the hospital and the doctor to start HRT but I want to avoid it. How can I cope with both arthritis when I need to keep warm and with hot flushes when I want to cool down?

You are doing everything you can to help yourself, with the alternative medicines and the dietary supplements. Some of the antidepressants have been found to be very good in low doses at stopping flushes (venlafaxine 37.5 mg at night) and can also be taken if you are on tamoxifen for breast cancer. Non-steroidal anti-inflammatory drugs can have side effects but like HRT, it has to be your evidence-based patient choice whether the quality of life from intermittently taking something to allow you to be pain free is better than being stiff and drenched in sweat!

(Editor's note: See Chapter 4 on HRT on page 43.)

Bladder and vaginal changes

Is there an increase in cystitis at the menopause?

Many women seem to suffer cystitis or similar symptoms around the time of the menopause. This is because the opening to the bladder neck shortens and can become dry, leaving it susceptible to infection.

I am 54 and going through the menopause. My main problem is bladder leakage when I sneeze or laugh and also when I'm at my aerobics class. It's really putting me

off going to the class. Are bladder problems caused by the menopause and what advice can you give me?

This is a very common problem, although the menopause itself may not be the direct cause. As you get older, the muscles in your pelvic floor become more lax, especially if you have had children. This results in a weakening in the muscles used to hold in urine and on exercise a small amount of urine leaks. It may also leak when pressure on the muscles is raised, by coughing or sneezing. If the problem is mild it can be helped by increasing the strength of the pelvic floor, through pelvic floor exercises. Ask your practice nurse for details. For more severe leakage, you may need an assessment. Possible treatments include medication or surgery. In any case, it is not a problem you simply have to put up with, so seek help.

I am 63 and a post-menopausal woman. For the past 18 months every so often I have had the feeling at the front of my vagina of wanting to pass water. I started noticing this when I ate fruit or foods containing citric acid, acetic acid or vinegar. I have stopped eating these foods and the problem has gone. I don't want to eliminate these foods forever. I suffer from irritable bowel syndrome and I have had to eliminate other foods because of IBS. I have used KY Jelly which has helped the dryness for quite a while. What can you suggest that will help me?

After the menopause, the level of oestrogen drops and your vagina gets dryer, less flexible and more alkaline. (An acidic vagina acts as an antiseptic to keep bacteria at bay.) This is called atrophic vaginitis. The same thing also happens to the bladder. It gets more irritable and sensitive to chemicals which have never bothered it before. You can also get more urinary tract infections, so it is always worth taking a urine specimen to your doctor to have it tested to exclude a low-grade infection that should be treated. Local oestrogen vaginal pessaries really help this symptom and need only to be used about twice a week, and have no long-term safety issues. It will also help your vaginal dryness. Alternatively, you could try an oral supplement of red clover.

Lately I have noticed what I think is a small amount of bladder weakness during the day, usually when my bladder is full. Not much and not every day. I don't have to keep going to the toilet frequently during the day. But during the night I need to go about every three hours and my bladder is always full. It is a real nuisance as I had started sleeping better than I was and now this keeps waking me up. I did wonder if I had an infection but I get no discomfort or any other symptoms. Is this a common problem at my age (59) and what can be done about it?

Yes, a number of things happen to our urinary systems after the menopause. Firstly, the lack of oestrogen makes the whole pelvic floor sag, so the bladder can slip down, or be dragged down as part of the uterus (womb) prolapsing. The good news is that pelvic floor exercises really help. Secondly, the opening of the bladder (the urethra) gapes more, letting in more bugs so leading to recurrent urinary tract infections (UTIs). Get a urinary specimen checked by your GP.

Also after sex, you may get infections as the vagina is dryer and more easily traumatised. Local oestrogen pessaries help both vaginal dryness and recurrent UTIs, without the breast cancer risks of systemic HRT. (For breast cancer risks and HRT see Appendix, see page 135.) Finally there is a whole crop of drugs that help with bladder muscle and its functions. You can also ask to be referred to a urogynaecology specialist clinic, where they can test for a weak bladder (stress incontinence) or an irritable bladder. Contact the Bladder and Bowel Foundation for more information.

I suffer from bladder weakness from time to time. I am too embarrassed to carry incontinence pads in my bag. Are there any discreet products you can recommend?

Like menstrual pads, incontinence pads have evolved over the years. They are now very discreet and comfortable and are designed for various levels of bladder weakness. TENA products range from a Mini (a pantyliner with odour control) to the Lady Extra Plus (with a higher absorption, double layers and a wide adhesive wrap for convenience). There are also various other products with absorption levels in-between. For women who prefer a garment rather than pads, TENA also has disposable pants, from the Discreet to the Super, which provide maximum security. The pants stay securely in place, have side-tears for easy removal and can be rolled up before disposal.

Please can you give me information about the causes of vaginal dryness.

Vaginal dryness is a common problem after the menopause because the lower level of the female hormone oestrogen results in the vaginal skin becoming thinner. The skin is more delicate and drier as there is less blood flow to it. Gynaecologists call this vaginal atrophy. Women may be aware of a generalised uncomfortable feeling during the day or it may be a problem mainly noticed during sexual intercourse. The dryness can be relieved by vaginal moisturisers and vaginal oestrogen cream or pessaries. Ordinary HRT (e.g. tablets or patches) on its own may not give enough relief from vaginal symptoms, but the two types of hormone treatment can be used together safely. General exercise, pelvic floor exercises and regular sex or masturbation are important for assisting with the blood flow to the vagina and pelvis.

Skin, hair and mouth problems

Sometimes I have a crawling feeling over my body. Is this a menopausal symptom?

What you are experiencing is a fairly common menopausal symptom called 'formication'. It does respond to HRT so mention it to your doctor.

I am 50 and I still have a period every few months. I have noticed some mottled pigmentation on my lower arms and on my neck. I am not on HRT. Could it be due to the menopause?

Changes in skin pigmentation can occur for a variety of reasons. These include skin diseases, hormonal causes (for example, when on the contraceptive pill or HRT), as a reaction to medicines or simply as part of the natural ageing process. The latter is the most likely cause, but a check with your GP will determine the cause in your case.

I am 49. I have itchy crawly skin, which is particularly bad a few days before a period. Having a shower (without shower gels) can bring on the itching. I am having my periods twice a month. I take flaxseed oil and soya supplements as well as drinking soya milk and eating soya-based foods.

As you get older, your skin gets dryer and more sensitive: try Aveeno moisturiser. Some women get very itchy in late pregnancy, and a similar phenomenon may be happening in the perimenopause. However, there are many other causes of itchy skin. There are illnesses that cause itching: liver, kidney or pancreas problems, as well as iron or vitamin B12 deficiencies, for example, so it may be worth asking your GP to do some blood tests. Be aware also that washing powders change their formulations. With hot flushes, you sweat more so more powder residue gets on your skin; you may be developing a washing powder allergy (change to a non-biological or hypoallergenic one). People can be allergic to soya-based foods. I itch when I try to eat tofu, so it may be your supplements: try a week without them and see if the itching stops!

I am 57. I am not on HRT but I take red clover tablets, as well as supplements including oils (containing evening primrose oil, avocado oil, hempseed and golden flax), and lutein. My main concern is my very dry skin,

particularly on my scalp, neck, body and eyes. What can I do about it? What pharmacy products are available?

Dry skin is often experienced by women during the perimeno-pause or menopause. This is due to a decrease in oestrogen and collagen production. The oil glands in the skin are not stimulated, resulting in dry skin and wrinkles. With age, the number of oil-producing sebaceous glands is reduced and the skin loses its ability to hold moisture. Dietary deficiencies in essential fatty acids and nutrients can also alter skin condition, but these are present in the supplements that you are taking. Moisturisers and emollients are available from pharmacies to reduce the dryness of skin; Aqueous cream is a cleanser that can be used instead of soap; E45 is a nourishing moisturis-er. Bath oils or additives in lukewarm water can be used for severe dry skin; products include Balneum, Balneum Plus and Emulsiderm. Hydromol Emollient can be used in the bath or in the shower, with Hydromol Ointment applied as a moistur-iser. All of the above products are available on prescription so it is worth requesting them from your GP if you are eligible for free medication.

What is the best way of relieving dry, itchy skin on my face and around my vagina?

The hormonal changes of the menopause often combine with general effects of ageing to cause dry itchy skin, generally and in the vagina. Skin on your face should respond well to using moisturisers regularly. Vaginal dryness occurs mainly because of a lack of oestrogen, often some time after the menopause, and is most easily treated with a local oestrogen cream or pessaries. Used at a very low dose on a regular basis, local oestrogens will improve vaginal dryness with few of the side effects of general HRT and can often be used by women who may not otherwise use HRT.

If you want to avoid oestrogen, you can buy vaginal moisturisers that don't contain hormones (e.g. Replens, Sylk, Astroglide). These need to be used on a more frequent basis than local oestrogens. If you decide to take general HRT, your skin may improve too.

What are age spots? Why do we get them?

Age spots are simply a discolouration of the skin, which becomes more common as we get older. They may occur anywhere, but are commonly seen on the arms and neck. They can be worsened by sitting in the sun and sometimes by the use of HRT or the contraceptive pill. They are harmless, but as with any skin changes you should seek the advice of your GP if you are concerned.

I seem to be getting more hair on my face. Could this be caused by the HRT I'm taking or is it my age (57)?

There is sometimes an increase in facial hair after the menopause, although this increase may be associated with decreased body hair and scalp hair follicles. It is more likely that increased facial hair is due to the general process of ageing rather than related to the HRT you are taking. However, if you are concerned, ask your doctor to change the type of HRT that you use.

Over the last five or six weeks I have noticed that a lot of hair is coming out on my hairbrush. My hairdresser tells me that my hair is thinning on top. Have you any suggestions about what I should do?

You should consider possible reasons for hair loss. These include washing hair with hard water, using chemical hair dyes and not eating a balanced diet. Low iron levels, for example, which can cause hair loss, could result in vitamin or mineral deficiencies. Some medical conditions also cause hair thinning, for example thyroid problems and stress. Your doctor will be able to help you work out if these are reasons for your hair loss and provide treatment. Alternatives ways to manage hair loss include a healthy lifestyle, with low stress, good diet and enough exercise and sleep, regular gentle hair oil massage to help improve local blood circulation and herbal or homeopathic treatment. Finally, it is important to remember that this can be part of the ageing process, and if there is a genetic or family tendency to hair loss, then there may be no effective treatment.

My gums are bleeding. Could this be due to the menopause? What can I do about it?

My dentist reckons he can tell when a woman is going though the menopause because her gums recede around this time. If your gums are actually bleeding then you do need to see your dentist, as you may have a low grade infection or gingivitis. Gums can also bleed if you are taking any anticoagulant medication (e.g. aspirin, warfarin, dipyridamole), or if you have a platelet abnormality. I have never seen a case of scurvy (vitamin C deficiency) but your gums are supposed to bleed with that too. If you have other signs of abnormal bleeding or bruising, see your GP for a blood test. A dental hygienist will advise you on gum care. A diet high in natural plant oestrogens (phytoestrogens) will help; try soya, tofu, lentils, beans, peas or red clover tablets.

I am 48, with a regular 28-day cycle so far. For the last year or so, I have been waking up at night with a very dry mouth over the last seven to ten days of each cycle. Could this be related to the menopause? Is there anything I can do to help it?

Women who suffer from pre-menstrual symptoms sometimes complain of dry mouth just before they get their periods. They also feel dehydrated and irritable, have problems sleeping and feel tired and lethargic. Reducing stress, taking light exercise, drinking water, eating healthily and sleeping well may help. You can also try over-the-counter products sold from pharmacies to relieve a dry mouth, like sugar-free pastilles or saliva-replacement gels. Dry mouth syndrome has been described as a menopausal symptom, but this is uncommon. It could be a result of psychological stress, perhaps due to the menopause itself, or other factors. Certain medicines can cause a dry mouth, so ask your doctor or pharmacist to check any medicines you are taking. If lifestyle changes don't help, then you should see a doctor for further advice.

Emotional symptoms

What are the most common psychological menopausal symptoms?

When women reach the menopause, they are often unsure about what is happening to them or why. They may experience problems concentrating, irritability, forgetfulness, a lack of motivation; an overreaction to minor upsets, feelings of sadness, bitterness, regret and panic, unexplained aggressiveness, mood swings, anxiousness or 'depression'. These symptoms are often due to hormonal fluctuations, which can be stressful in themselves, combined with external pressures (such as caring for elderly parents or work or relationship issues) and internal conflicts (for example 'this isn't what I expected').

I am 45 and I had a hysterectomy two years ago. I still have my ovaries. My main problem is depression. I have tried different types of anti-depressants, which have not helped. What can you suggest?

Although you still have your ovaries, you may be experiencing a menopause that affects your mood. Speak to your GP or practice nurse about a hormone assay. The emotional response after a hysterectomy varies widely and depends on several factors including feelings about the operation, symptom relief, timing, whether you have completed your family and whether you have supportive relationships. Some feelings may be an expression of grief for a lost aspect of yourself or the life you had hoped for. Regular exercise, stress management and natural remedies can help, although it is most important to find someone you can confide in, such as a relative, friend, or counsellor/psychologist. A support group where you can learn from the experiences of others as well as share your own, can also be helpful.

My GP has suggested that I consult a counsellor about my anxiety. What will a consultation involve?

Many people find the prospect of a first consultation daunting because they don't know what to expect. A meeting usually lasts about an hour and the information shared is confidential.

The counsellor will invite you to talk about your difficulties in some detail to understand better how you view them, and will then share his/her psychological knowledge with you to try to help you make sense of what you are experiencing. If this feels helpful, this would form the basis of subsequent meetings, which may include a recommended package of care. You would be involved in putting this together, as a way of helping you to move forward.

I experience terrible mood swings which are affecting my life and I should like to see a counsellor. How can I find a counsellor in my area and in what way could they help me?

Concerns around mood swings tend to be addressed in medical settings by interested GPs, specialist clinics, nurses, community pharmacists and possibly nutritionists. Very few include a counsellor or psychologist as an integrated part of their service. No specific training for counsellors includes the menopause, although most current practitioners are actually women at mid-life. However, many counsellors are trained in stress management and can draw on these skills to help you understand any issues associated with mood swings, for example feelings of resentment or bitterness, and/or unrealised hopes and expectations. They can also help you to find coping strategies to counter some of the negative impact, through, for example, finding appropriate ways of prioritising your own health and sense of wellbeing. Local practitioners can be found either through your GP or accrediting bodies such as the British Psychological Society, the British Association for Counselling and Psychotherapy and the United Kingdom Council for Psychotherapy.

I'm 52 and I've started getting panic attacks. I've heard that they can come with the menopause. Is this true and what's the best way to cope with them?

Erratic hormonal fluctuations can produce symptoms similar to those experienced in panic attacks. Both involve an intense fear of losing control. Although the menopause is a healthy life change, panic attacks are not and help is available.

The risk of a panic attack increases with the number of negative life events, such as illness or death, experiences in the past year, and sometimes the meaning attributed to them. Often, after an initial attack, there is fear of a repeat.

Understanding that attacks are not in reality life-threatening helps some people, as does recognising an attack is coming. Deep breathing exercises help to reduce the intensity of symptoms; visualising relaxing images reduces self-consciousness and abates symptoms; calming self-talk also helps, for example 'I am not dying, I have experienced this before, everything will be alright' and listening to a relaxation tape or music.

I'm in my 40s. I'm going through the menopause and am continually worried about everything. I know that I'm more irritable than usual. It's difficult to cope with the demands of a job, a son of 18 taking exams this year and a widower father who finds it difficult to look after himself. I don't want to go on HRT. Do you have you any suggestions?

The menopause involves psychological as well as physical changes. From what you say, you seem to view it as a negative experience, and this in itself can affect your mood. Your son's exams represent a passport to a new and independent life, and some of your underlying worries may also be around how you will be affected when he leaves. Practical support for your father may be available from agencies like social services, friends, neighbours or community organisations – he may even be more capable than you think. Like many women, you seem to put your own needs last. Clear communication of these could go some way towards getting support and reducing irritability. Dietary changes can also make a big difference (such as cutting out caffeine and alcohol, eating plenty of fruit and vegetables), as can taking more exercise. Acupuncture, aromatherapy, Alexander technique and yoga, are all enjoyable as well as health enhancing and relaxing. All influence the way you think and feel.

I'm at my wit's end with my body. Sometimes I'm on top of everything, then suddenly I can't control my emotions. I'm very reluctant to go on HRT or anything medical, as I feel that I will get over this with exercise and diet. I have had acupuncture, which has helped. What advice can you give me?

Many women are turning to exercise, diet and a variety of relaxation enhancing techniques, all of which can positively affect emotions and help you believe that this time of life can include looking and feeling good. Specifically, activities such as an exercise programme can help, as will developing new and creative interests. Although it may feel like it at times, our minds, thoughts and feelings are not separate from our bodies. Feelings are affected both by life events and by how you think about your situation. You may be associating the menopause with negative aspects of ageing, unattractiveness and loss of social power. Developing alternative more realistic views can positively influence how you value yourself. Reviewing your lifestyle, the balance between work and leisure, between meeting your needs and pleasing other people, all impact on how you feel. Activities such as yoga, Tai chi, meditation and relaxation exercises (all of which control your breathing) can be beneficial. Most important perhaps is keeping the lines of communication open with those to whom you feel close, letting them know what you are experiencing and how they may help, and also developing new interests.

I am suffering from unexplainable stress at present. Can the menopause increase stress? I feel sleepy during the day. I checked with my GP, but she didn't give me a satisfactory reply.

Fatigue (severe tiredness) is a common menopausal symptom. It can put pressure on your work, home life and relationships. This adds to stress, making you less able to cope with the demands of your changing body at this time of life, for example sleep-disturbing night sweats. Cigarette smoking, sugar and caffeine tend to diminish energy after an initial buzz, whereas fresh fruit and vegetables supply healthy support. Rest, relaxation and enjoyable leisure activities help you keep active and mentally alert. Regular exercise, meditation, breathing exercises, yoga and Tai chi can help relieve built-up tension and have a calming effect on the mind. Self-affirming positive thoughts maintain self-confidence and prevent self-criticism. The strong interaction between mind and body means negative thoughts can make menopause more stressful but communicating with loved ones or a good laugh creates neurochemical changes that counter the effects of stress, relieving muscular tension, improving breathing, and regulating the heart beat.

Can stress management help menopausal symptoms? If so, what advice can you give me?

Several studies[3, 4] have linked hot flushes to increased stress, although optimism and self-esteem are also factors. Keep a flush or hassle diary. Then take responsibility and get active: take a few deep breaths in, then slow breaths out – this is calming, prevents you getting too 'wound up' and can help you anticipate triggers, for example for hot flushes, and so reduce them. Having good relationships, talking with others and being assertive about your needs help, as does being spontaneous and having a laugh! Much of stress is to do with perception: if you can view your situation more positively, your stressors (including menopausal symptoms) become more manageable. Set aside some time for yourself and to meet with friends; consider your diet and incorporate physical activities such as exercises meditation, yoga or massage – the key is to find meaning and pleasure!

Weight and digestive problems

I am 54 years old and my periods are erratic. At the moment, I feel alright and don't seem to have any menopausal symptoms but I am overweight and worried that my weight may give me problems with the menopause in the future. Have you found this?

If you are overweight you might be prone to suffer more with hot flushes and sweats. Also, if you decide to use HRT, patches and gels may be absorbed less efficiently. Being overweight and reaching menopausal years gives rise to a greater risk of heart disease. The recommendation is to lose weight by taking aerobic weight-bearing exercise two to three times a week. Eat a low-sugar, low-fat diet, cutting down on starchy carbohydrates.

I have never had a weight problem before and now I put weight on just looking at food despite going to the gym three to four times a week. Another problem is when my

periods start going erratic. If I miss a period for three to four months I find it hard to know whether my body feels normal or not. I seem to get all sorts of aches and pains and then just when I think my periods have stopped for good along comes another one! How do you know when to be worried or not?

This could be the early stages of menopause, often described as the perimenopause. Every woman is individual and for some this stage may last a couple of years, until her periods finally stop completely. Weight management is important at all ages, but especially in your 40s and 50s when it can be too easy to allow the pounds to creep on, almost without noticing. Weight loss is not always easy but a sustained pattern of healthy eating along with regular exercise should stop it piling on. See your practice nurse or GP for sensible advice about healthy eating, as well as finding out about the potential effects of the menopause. Finally, if you are worried about your health, do not hesitate to make an appointment with your GP – GPs are there for that very reason and should never make you feel that you might be wasting their time.

Can you tell me about bloating in the post-menopause? Is it a menopausal symptom? I am not on HRT.

Bloating is a sensation experienced by an individual. It cannot be measured scientifically. Many post-menopausal women complain of bloating, although it is not specifically a menopausal symptom. Bloating can be due to any or all of the following:

- Weight gain.
- Altered fat distribution. The natural changes in hormone levels cause fat to be redistributed from the hips to the waist. This causes loss of waist narrowing and may feel like bloating.
- Fluid retention from a variety of causes.
- Slower movement through the bowel with gaseous distension.

The recommendation is to eat a healthy balanced diet, reduce your caffeine intake and exercise regularly. If problems persist, see your GP.

Chapter 3

Osteoporosis

Osteoporosis literally means 'porous bones'. If you have osteoporosis, your bones are much more fragile than normal and can break (fracture) easily. One in two women and one in five men over the age of 50 in the UK will break a bone, mainly due to osteoporosis.

Bones are constantly changing, so old bone is regularly broken down and replaced by new bone. This process of renewal is called 'cell turnover'. If you have healthy bones, your rate of bone breakdown is equal to the rate of formation, so your bone mass stays fairly constant.

As you get older, the rate at which your bones break down increases and exceeds the rate at which they are formed. If you have osteoporosis, bone is lost much faster than new bone is laid down. This leaves your bones much more likely to break, especially in the wrist, hip and spine. Spinal fractures are often responsible for the curved spine, loss of height and back pain that some people develop in later life.

Men and women start to experience bone loss after the age of 35. However, oestrogen plays a part in keeping bones healthy so women are more prone to the condition as they get older. After the menopause, a lack of oestrogen makes your bones weaker and more brittle so they may break more easily.

The diagnosis of osteoporosis is based on the measurement of your bone density (a bone density scan). Low bone density may lead to an increased risk of fractures. The most common method for assessing bone density is a dual energy x-ray absorptiometry (DEXA) scan, which measures your bone strength and can diagnose osteoporosis and your future risk of fractures. DEXA scans usually scan some bones in your lower spine and one hip, but sometimes in your forearm or heel. The results will show how your bone density compares with the average bone density of a young healthy adult. It is expressed in terms of standard deviation (SD) and you are given a T score. A Z score, which compares your results with someone of your own age, is also calculated.

When bone density in either the hip or spine is measured, people are placed in three categories: normal; osteopaenia (slightly below average); and osteoporosis. Depending on the scan results, you may need to consider treatment to boost your bone mineral density.

Ultrasound scanning, usually of the heel bone, wrist or finger, can't assess bone density or diagnose osteoporosis. Biochemical bone markers gauge how quickly bone is being broken down, but can't also be used to diagnose osteoporosis.

There are questions and answers on looking after your bones in chapter 6.

***

My 54-year-old friend gets hot flushes and has osteoporosis. I am the same age, but I haven't had any hot flushes yet. I would like to know what could put me at risk of osteoporosis.

All women vary, although most women go through the menopause between the ages of 45 and 55. Around 25 per cent of women sail through the menopause without experiencing any of the associated vasomotor symptoms, such as hot flushes and night sweats. So in your case, either you are yet to start the menopause (in which case you are still probably having roughly regular monthly periods) or you are within the group of lucky women who will not be troubled by menopausal symptoms (such as hot flushes).

Risk factors for osteoporosis include:

- Age.
- Being female.
- Being Caucasian.
- Having a small body frame, especially if this is due to anorexia or bulimia or over-exercising.
- Menopause, as the hormone oestrogen helps to maintain bone mineral density.
- Family history. Women whose mothers have had a hip fracture are at a higher risk of fracture themselves and should be advised to see their doctor for assessment.
- Lifestyle. This includes low levels of physical exercise, cigarette smoking and high alcohol intake. The last two are toxic to bone cells.
- Poor nutrition. It is important to remember that a balanced protein and carbohydrate intake is as important as adequate calcium intake.
- Disease states that are known to cause osteoporosis include

hyperthyroidism (an overactive thyroid), hyperparathy-roidism (an overactive parathyroid gland), diabetes mel-litus, amenorrhoea (lack of periods before menopause), coeliac disease (gluten intolerance), inflammatory bowel disease, alcoholism and rheumatoid arthritis.

- Some drugs that are known to cause osteoporosis include glucocorticoids (anti-inflammatories), anticonvulsants (for epilepsy) and heparin (for blood clotting).

If you are worried that you have a medical condition or are taking any drug treatment that increases your osteoporosis risk, please discuss this with your doctor who will advise on appropriate action. From the lifestyle point of view, it is impor-tant that you take daily weight-bearing exercise (such as brisk walking), stop smoking, drink less alcohol and have a good bal-anced diet, including calcium- and vitamin D-rich foods.

(Editor's note: Vasomotor symptoms are symptoms caused by the irregular function of the part of the brain that controls body heat.)

Please can you give me information on weight-bearing exercise for both the prevention and treatment of oste-oporosis. Which types of exercise are weight-bearing? How often and for how long should they be carried out to gain adequate benefit?

Physical exercise, where you are active and on the move, has been found to help prevent osteoporosis. However, it is not known how much exercise everyone should do. Some US re-search[5] showed that when 375 adults acted on healthy lifestyle advice (to include good diet and weight-bearing exercise), this helped to reduce their risk factors for osteoporosis and fractures (broken bones). On average, in this study each person had two strength training sessions and around 130 minutes of aerobic exercise per week. People who took part in this study had good intentions. However, though they continued with a good diet, unfortunately they took less exercise with time.

Aerobic exercises can be any form of exercise that makes your heart pump, but it is important not to over-exert yourself suddenly. Examples of weight-bearing exercise are brisk walking for 20 minutes every day, or weekly aerobic classes or dance exercise classes, where you built up your exercise routine slowly.

Some simple advice on weight-bearing exercise:
1) The younger you start exercising the better. When you are young your bones are most responsive to mechanical stimuli (the weight your bones carry whilst active) which in turn makes your bone stronger.
2) Select exercises that are dynamic and high-impact. You may wish to get advice from a fitness expert at the gym. Examples are jumping for the lower parts of your body and racquet sports for the upper parts of your body.
3) Try exercising the specific bone regions you want to strengthen, as the bone response to mechanical loads is most effective at the bone area being exercised.
4) Exercising briefly yet often is known to be effective.
5) It is very important to continue exercise and keep active and mobile (on the move) as you age to prevent bone loss and reduce the risk of falls.

Following these steps will help to promote bone health at all ages, and may reduce your risk of a fracture by improving bone mass and size during youth, while reducing age-related bone loss and the risk of falls in adulthood.

What general health, nutrition and supplements advice would you give to a high-powered career woman in her early 50s with the following profile: hysterectomy at 35, underactive thyroid for the past five years (100 micrograms thyroxine daily), very active (tennis, rowing, walked the marathon), recently diagnosed with osteopaenia?

An early hysterectomy and your recently diagnosed osteopaenia (thinning of the bones) give us cause to look at your calcium intake carefully. The great news is that walking and tennis are two of the best exercises you can do for maintaining strong bones. In terms of calcium, you need to be eating at least 700 milligrams per day. Try to ensure that you are including a serving of dairy food at least three times each day (milk, yoghurts, milk puddings, cheese etc). Other good sources of calcium include canned fish, breads, baked beans and seeds and nuts. Smoking and heavy alcohol intake promote thinning of the bones. The phytoestrogens contained in soya, soya products and linseed may help to protect bones, so eating these regularly will also help. Try using Burgen bread, canned soya beans in casseroles or salads and toasting linseed to use on breakfast cereals or in baking.

Chapter 4

HRT

(Hormone Replacement Therapy)

HRT is the main medical treatment for menopausal symptoms. The oestrogen in HRT relieves symptoms such as hot flushes, night sweats, vaginal symptoms, urinary frequency and urgency and mood swings. HRT also prevents osteoporosis and reduces the risk of spine and hip fractures.

If you have had a hysterectomy and therefore have no uterus, you need to take oestrogen-only HRT. If you have a uterus, you need to take progesterone as well as oestrogen, to protect your uterine (womb) lining (called the endometrium) and reduce your risk of endometrial cancer.

There are three types of combined oestrogen and progesterone HRT. With sequential combined (cyclical combined) HRT, you take the oestrogen continuously and the progesterone for 10 to 14 days each month to mimic your natural hormone cycle. This usually causes a withdrawal bleed. Continuous combined (also called period-free or no-bleed) HRT, which involves taking both oestrogen and progesterone daily, is prescribed to women who haven't had a natural period for 12 months. Long-cycle HRT gives a withdrawal bleed every three months.

Oestrogen-only HRT is available in the form of oral tablets, implants, patches, skin gels and vaginal preparations. Forms of progesterone (or progestogen, the synthetic form of progesterone) are available as oral tablets, capsules, in patches with oestrogen, pessaries, vaginal gel and an intrauterine-system (IUS).

As Dr Mark Porter wrote in an article for The Menopause Exchange,[6] 'HRT is like wearing a dress. What suits one woman won't do a thing for another.' So, the type, form and dose need to be tailored to each woman's needs.

The decision about whether or not to go on HRT needs to be made with your doctor. Think of the decision as a pair of scales – weighing up the benefits (pros) on one side against the risks (cons) on the other. You need to get the balance right.

Before making a decision, you should consider your age, the type and severity of your symptoms and how your symptoms affect your life – in other words, how they affect your home life, your relationships and your work (if you work). Then you should think about the benefits that you would gain from using or taking HRT (e.g. the reduction in your menopausal symptoms).

Your doctor will tell you if there are any reasons why you can't take HRT (e.g. breast cancer or venous thromboembolism (blood clots in the legs)). These reasons are called 'contraindications'.

You and your doctor should then discuss your personal risks if you take HRT by considering your own medical history and your family history of certain medical conditions.

Finally, you can weigh up your own pros and cons for taking HRT, bearing in mind your personal preference. When you make a decision, your doctor will bear in mind the current guidelines on taking HRT, which change over time as results from new research studies are published.

***

I am 54 and have been using HRT patches for a couple of years. My mother-in-law keeps telling me that in her day menopausal women managed without any medical treatment – they just got on with it and it never did them any harm. Is she right? Is HRT unnecessary and should I just be accepting my symptoms as a natural part of life?

Every generation is different. The field of HRT has advanced enormously in the last 10 to 15 years, and the fact that we can now take a treatment for those awful menopausal symptoms, which for most women is safe and convenient, is a medical advance most of us appreciate. Only you know how your symptoms were affecting your life before HRT; if they were mild and not too troublesome, maybe you could manage fine without HRT. If however, they were moderate or severe and were affecting your home and work life, and assuming you discussed the benefits and risks for you with your doctor, then why not continue to accept some relief? Every woman is different and for some HRT will be a positive benefit. As for your mother-in-law, well, maybe menopause is a bit like giving birth – you forget how awful it can be!

Which HRT products have natural ingredients?

This depends on what you call 'natural'. HRT is a medicine that has been extensively researched and manufactured in laboratories. It mimics natural oestrogen, so is described as 'natural' rather than synthetic (for example, the contraceptive pill is synthetic). The ingredients of some HRT products are derived from plant extracts, e.g. those containing oestradiol, whilst conjugated oestrogens are derived from animal extracts. However, the clinical effect of 'natural HRT' and 'synthetic HRT' is considered to be similar for most women, as long as we understand that 'natural HRT' means oestradiol based, and 'synthetic' means conjugated. Occasionally, there is a medical reason why one particular product should be used or avoided.

My doctor says that I have to take progesterone as well as oestrogen in my HRT. Why is this?

If you have not had a hysterectomy, it is essential that you do not take oestrogen therapy on its own, but use a combined oestrogen/progestogen form of HRT. This is because oestrogen causes the uterine (womb) lining to thicken if used on its own. If allowed to develop for a long period of time, this could eventually be harmful to your uterus. The progestogen will prevent this from happening. It does not matter if you use monthly or continuous HRT, the progestogen is still important. Of course, if you have had a hysterectomy, this problem need not concern you!

Do I have to bleed on HRT?

Obviously this question does not apply to the 20 per cent of women who have had a hysterectomy (their uterus removed).

For the rest, it depends on where you are in the menopause, and what you want to do, but the short answer is 'no'.

Women who are a year post-menopause (no period for one year) can take 'continuous combined' regimes where they don't bleed. Women in the perimenopause (who are still having periods) can take either 'sequential HRT', where they will have withdrawal bleeds, or can use the Mirena coil (levonorgestrel intra-uterine system) inserted as the progestogenic part of HRT. This IUS has huge advantages as it is an extremely good contraceptive (women in the perimenopause still need to use contraception), and it stops their periods too. Then you can add in an oestrogen of your choice in tablet, gel or patch form. There is the minor inconvenience and discomfort of getting a Mirena fitted, but then it is in for four years so should see you through the menopause. Discuss this with your GP or family planning clinic.

My doctor has suggested that I have a Mirena fitted as the progesterone part of HRT. Please can you give me information on it.

The Mirena is an intra-uterine system (IUS). It has been available in the UK for some years, primarily licensed for contraception and for women who suffer from heavy bleeding. Mirena is different to other IUDs as it also contains the progestogen levonorgestrel, which is embedded within the device. The progestogen content provides further drug treatment, in addition to the effect of having a physical device inserted within the uterus. The Mirena is also licensed to be used as the progestogen component of HRT for up to four years. It can be inserted at any time in a woman who is not bleeding menstrually or during the last days of menstruation or withdrawal bleeding.

If you are prescribed a Mirena as part of your HRT, you will be prescribed oestrogen separately. The progestogen's role in HRT is to protect the uterine (womb) lining. Generally, the Mirena is a good choice as part of HRT in cases of bleeding problems or where progestogen sensitivity causes worse side effects when progestogen is taken as a tablet or patch than when it is used as the Mirena.

Why do I have to pay two prescription charges for HRT?

It does seem unfair, but in the UK if a prescribed course of products contains two or more medications on different days (in this case oestrogen and progestogen), then two charges are made. It does not matter that the two products are actually in only one tablet or patch. Women using oestrogen and progestogen throughout the month ('no bleed' treatment) pay only one charge, because the treatment is the same throughout the month. (Just remember outside the UK you would be paying a whole lot more!)

What health checks will be carried out before I go on HRT? How often and for how long will I be monitored once I start HRT?

Before starting HRT, you will be asked about your problems. You should be weighed and measured, your blood pressure checked, and you will be asked about smoking, alcohol, diet and exercise. You will have blood tests or an internal examination only if you have a problem needing further investigation.

You will be asked about your risks of osteoporosis, blood clots, heart disease, stroke and breast cancer. This will include details of your family history to look for inherited factors. If necessary to make a decision, you will be offered a bone density measurement, clotting screen or mammogram. These aren't done routinely.

You will be reviewed after two or three months to assess the effectiveness of the HRT prescription you were given. It is recommended that further review occur at least annually. At this time, your blood pressure will usually be checked; you will only have more tests if there are good reasons to do so.

How soon will HRT work? What benefits should I look out for?

HRT is prescribed for symptoms caused by reduced oestrogen levels. The benefit expected is therefore reduced severity of these symptoms. Women without symptoms won't be aware of any benefit. Ideally, patients are given a dose and route of delivery that will restore their previous state of wellbeing, although a compromise may be necessary. Generally we start with low doses and an adjustment may be needed before full benefit is felt. Some improvement should be felt within two weeks, although flushes may take six to eight weeks to recede. Vaginal improvement can continue for up to 12 months.

When is the right time of day to take HRT and with what should you take HRT? Are there any supplements that might interact with or affect it?

It actually doesn't matter that much what time of day you take HRT, but it is best to be consistent. Most women take the tablets with breakfast in the morning, as actually remembering to take any long-term medication is the tricky bit. Similarly, women use the gels on getting up. I had one 30-year-old with a premature menopause who split up her gel into morning and evening, as she got a headache using the full dose all together. Patches you have to write in your diary to remind you to change them.

Calcium and vitamin D supplements can block absorption of other tablets, so take these with your lunch or supper, but not with other medication.

How do you know if you are through the menopause if you are on HRT?

If you start HRT before your periods finally stop you will not know the actual date that your menopause occurs. The average age of menopause is about 51 years and by the age of 54 years, 80 per cent of women are through the menopause. If you are on HRT, the only reason you may need to know the time of your menopause is to assess whether or not you need to continue contraception. In such cases, women usually continue using some form of contraception until about 55 yrs of age.

How do I know if I'm fertile if I'm on HRT?

This is a problem for younger women on HRT. The only way to determine fertility is to stop your HRT for a washout period of about two months. You would then have a blood test to calculate the level of a hormone called follicle stimulating hormone (FSH). The amount of this hormone is generally low, but it then rises with the menopause. It is therefore generally a good indicator of menopausal status. The general rule for continuing with contraception whilst not on HRT is for two years if your periods stop under the age of 50 and one year if they stop after the age of 50.

Can any form of HRT act as a contraceptive as well?

This is a common misconception. None of the HRT preparations will act as contraceptives as well. The hormones in the contraceptive pill are synthetic (e.g. ethinyloestradiol) and are given in much higher amounts than the hormones in HRT to suppress ovulation. The majority of HRT preparations contain oestradiol, which is the same as the oestrogen your ovaries secrete each month when you are menstruating. The amount of oestrogen in HRT is enough to control your menopausal symptoms but it is not intended to suppress ovulation as well. A woman who is on HRT but is at risk of becoming pregnant will need to use contraception at the same time.

I am 47 and taking HRT for hot flushes and night sweats. I have been told that we must use condoms. Why do we need to do this? Won't the HRT act in the same way as the contraceptive pill?

For many women, the menopause marks the time when contraception is no longer required. However, in the early stages of menopause, it is still possible to get pregnant, even on HRT. If you are under 50 and not on HRT you should continue to use contraception for a further two years. If you start HRT whilst still having periods, however irregular, your last actual period will be masked so you will not know when to stop contraception. It is generally advised that to be safe you should continue using contraception until the age of about 54 yrs. HRT is not a contraceptive.

(Editor's note: The general rule for continuing with contraception whilst not on HRT is to use it for one year if periods stop after the age of 50.)

Will HRT improve a woman's sex life?

If your sex life was fine before the menopause, it is likely to be fine afterwards. However, some women do experience sexual problems after the menopause. Whether HRT will help these problems depends on their causes. For example, painful sexual intercourse is often related to hormone levels and can be successfully treated with HRT. However, other problems, such as loss of libido, can be related to hormones, a psychological/emotional trigger or be due to both, and success of treatment with HRT depends on which element predominates. A loss of libido that is secondary to hormonal deficiency can be very successfully treated with HRT, the drug Livial (tibolone) or the hormone testosterone, but psychosexual causes of a loss of libido cannot be treated with these drugs.

I would like information on oestrogen implants, their insertion and their advantages and disadvantages over other forms of HRT.

Oestrogen implants have been used to treat menopausal symptoms for over 50 years. The implants in use today have 17 beta oestradiol (a type of oestrogen) contained within a cholesterol base. Your doctor will decide what dose you should have after taking a medical history. Women with a uterus should also have a progestogen prescribed when an oestrogen implant is used.

Insertion is a relatively simple procedure, and involves the placing of the oestradiol pellet into the fat layer of your abdominal wall, after an incision is made using an instrument called a trocar (which is a sharply pointed steel rod covered with a tight fitting cylindrical tube, more generally used by doctors to drain or extract fluid from a body cavity). This allows a 'no touch' technique under a local anaesthetic and you should only feel minor discomfort.

One advantage of having oestrogen implants is that you benefit from pure, natural oestradiol, without having to remember to take tablets or use patches on certain days of the week. This form of administration is useful for younger patients, women who can't take tablets and when there is a need to avoid using the liver too much. A testosterone implant may be inserted at the same time as the oestrogen implant in women who have gone through the menopause and have a loss of libido.

The disadvantages include the need for special equipment, a possible risk of wound infection and difficulty in removing the oestrogen implant if side effects occur. There is the need to take progestogen in women with an intact uterus, and this may need to be continued for many months after a decision is made to stop oestrogen implants.

To avoid the risk of tachyphylaxis (where levels of oestrogen in the blood system are too high as a result of too many oestrogen implants over time), women are usually required to have an oestradiol blood test two weeks prior to attending for an implant. The oestrogen implant will only be given if oestradiol levels in the blood are within the safe range and are low and patients complain of symptoms. It is important to note that oestradiol blood tests are not useful when women take oestrogen tablets, as blood levels vary and don't correlate with the dose in tablet form that is being taken.

I am 41 years old and I have been on HRT for approximately six weeks. I am on oestrogen-only HRT having had a total hysterectomy. Due to high blood pressure and type 2 diabetes, which is well controlled, I have to be carefully monitored by my GP. I still get hot flushes and vaginal dryness. Can herbal remedies be used to combat these symptoms or will I need to increase my dose of HRT or use a local vaginal oestrogen cream? Can oestrogen-only HRT help with libido? If not, would I need to take added testosterone due to the loss of both my ovaries?

HRT is essential following a total hysterectomy and removal of the ovaries at an early age and should be continued until about the age of 51 when a natural menopause would be expected. Six weeks of treatment is not long, and an assessment is usually made after three months. Oestrogen cream or pessaries are excellent for vaginal dryness and can be safely used alongside oral HRT if necessary.

Clinicians judge the effectiveness of HRT according to the improvement in symptoms and any side effects an individual may notice. The dose and route of your current HRT can easily be adjusted to improve symptom control. It is probably better to do this first, rather than add in herbal remedies at this stage, as being relatively young you may need higher doses of oestrogen.

Oestrogen by itself doesn't increase sex drive, but by improving unpleasant symptoms and sleep, can make sexual relations more desirable. Testosterone does increase sex drive and may be added to standard HRT to replace the testosterone that the ovaries would have made.

I had some Zoff adhesive remover wipes at home for removing plaster marks and it seems to be very good at removing the gum that's left on my skin when I take off my HRT patch. Is it alright to use it for this? Can you recommend anything else?

Zoff is indeed helpful at removing the marks left behind by patches. However, in most cases, the mark (usually minor) can be removed simply by using baby oil. This is kinder to your skin in the long term. If the patches leave a red, sore area after removal, then you may be allergic to the adhesive in the patch. You should seek advice from your doctor or nurse.

I am diabetic and on insulin. I have terrible hot flushes and still have periods. Can diabetics take HRT? If so, are there any types that are best for them?

Diabetic women certainly can take HRT, and it may help to improve insulin sensitivity and control. As you are still having periods, you would need both oestrogen and progestogen to protect the uterus (womb) lining. The choice is complicated by the fact that the various types of oestrogen and progestogen differ in their impact on cholesterol and insulin. It may therefore be worth seeing a menopause specialist, who can look at your overall situation and advise on which combination may be best suited to your risk profile.

Please can you tell me about thinning hair. Are there any forms of HRT or particular HRT products that are hair and scalp friendly?

Most women, like men, with age develop widening partings and thinning of the hair all over the scalp. This is normal. It actually starts in the teens or early twenties, and by the age of 50 over half of all women have thinning hair. After the menopause, thinning of the hair can be more pronounced. Hair can also become thin at the front, which is similar to the male pattern. This is because the hair follicles are responding in exactly the same way as in balding men to the testosterone in the blood. All women have testosterone; this is perfectly normal. The balding doesn't mean that a woman has more testosterone; it simply means that the hair follicles on her scalp are over-sensitive, and it is thought that this is probably an inherited situation. The other explanation often given is that with loss of oestrogen during the menopause in women, the usual balance between oestrogen and testosterone in the blood is altered, with testosterone becoming higher as compared with oestrogen. What is important to understand is that the hair will thin only to a certain extent and then stop. There is no need to worry that you will become completely bald.

HRT, depending on the type, can affect your hair. If you are taking HRT containing progestogen, ask your doctor for the type of progestogen which is less similar to male hormones and which may therefore be better for women with hair loss.

It is important to remember that other causes for thinning hair in women include

- Age (most old people have thinner hair than when they were young).
- Heredity (some people are programmed to have thin hair, particularly as they get older).
- Hormone disorders (particularly underactive thyroid gland).
- Medicines.
- Iron deficiency (most likely in women who are vegetarians).
- Severe mental stress (such as bereavement), two to three months previously.
- Severe physical illness of any sort two to three months previously (particularly a high fever or severe infection – the hair grows again when the body has fully recovered).
- Childbirth (it's common to shed a lot of hair for one to six months after childbirth, but this usually grows again afterwards).
- Systemic lupus erythematosus (SLE), a disease affecting the connective tissue.
- Damage from hair bleaches and relaxers, which can damage the hair so that it becomes 'soapy' in texture and breaks off (Afro-Caribbean hair is especially vulnerable).

My friend and I both want to come off HRT. I'm taking tablets. She's using patches. What is the best way to come off them?

Don't stop suddenly as you'll get all your symptoms back. Come down slowly over about three months and stabilise at each new level before you go lower. Patches can be cut (before you take the backing off using a clean pair of nail scissors) to reduce the dose slowly. First month: cut patches into two-thirds/one-third. Use a two-thirds patch for four days then use up two of the one-third patches for the next four days (so you have reduced the HRT by one third). Second month: cut patch in half. Use half a patch for four days and the other half for four days. Third month: depending on how you are feeling do one-quarter patches or one-third. Fourth month: no more patches if you did one quarter last month and were OK, or do another low-dose month if you still have symptoms.

Tablets are more difficult as there is less flexibility. They are so small that they are really difficult to cut in half, let alone quarters. Ask your GP if it is the lowest dose available; you may be on 2 mg oestradiol preparations, when there are 1 mg preparations. Once on 1 mg oestradiol, try one to three months on half a tab, then one quarter of a tablet if you can manage it and then stop.

(Editor's note: Please speak to your doctor before coming off HRT.)

Should women stop HRT when they have surgery?

This is a controversial question. The safe answer is to check with your surgeon and anaesthetist when your surgery is planned, because they may well refuse to anaesthetise you if you have not stopped HRT. It partly depends on the anaesthetic: general or local. For a quick local anaesthetic (say to take off an ingrowing toe nail) there can be no rationale to stop as you'll be limping out of the clinic within 15 minutes. The situation is different if you have a general anaesthetic. HRT increases the risk of a deep vein thrombosis (blood clot) and, unfortunately major surgery does too, especially surgery on your hips or knees (anything that stops your legs pumping the blood back). So you are in for a double risk. Usually HRT is stopped six weeks before surgery and not restarted until you are fully mobile again (often a month post-op). To prevent hot flushes returning you need to wean yourself off HRT slowly over at least six weeks before you stop (i.e. three weeks on half a dose, three weeks on a quarter dose, then stop).

(Editor's note: Stopping HRT over three months is ideal but in this case you may have to do it more quickly).

Could you advise me whether it's possible that, whilst I was on HRT, I could have gone through the menopause 'behind the scenes' as it were and didn't experience any hot flushes etc, and now I've come off it, I've bypassed all those nasty symptoms?

HRT will help you through the time that you experience menopausal symptoms. Most women will take HRT for a while and then try without, to see if their symptoms have gone. If they have, then you have successfully 'bypassed' your symptoms. Some women get a few symptoms back when they stop HRT. If your symptoms return and are moderate or severe, you may need to restart the HRT, if appropriate.

(Editor's note: Vasomotor symptoms have an approximately 50 per cent chance of recurring when HRT is discontinued, independent of age and duration of use.[7])

I am thinking of going on HRT. Will it affect my contact lenses?

HRT itself shouldn't have an effect on contact lenses. However, around the time of the menopause, some women experience dry eyes, which can affect lens wearing. Also, the ageing process itself continues despite the use of HRT and some changes may occur to your eyes at this time. It is always worthwhile having an up-to-date eye examination to ensure your current lens prescription is accurate.

Does HRT affect blood pressure?

The scientific evidence has shown that HRT doesn't increase blood pressure for most women. A very small number of women react unusually to conjugated equine oestrogens (for example Premarin), with a blood pressure increase. (Conjugated equine oestrogens are a type of oestrogen used in HRT and are obtained from mares' urine.) A check after three months will show whether or not a blood pressure increase has occurred. Be aware that blood pressure can go up at this time of life for all sorts of other reasons and ought to be monitored. High blood pressure is primarily a risk factor for stroke. If raised it may alter the risk analysis and decision about whether or not to continue to take HRT.

I have varicose veins. Is it safe for me to take HRT? If so, what form of HRT would be best?

Everyone has varicose veins. But they get worse as we get older, because we have stood on our legs for longer. The little valves in the veins that help the venous blood get back to the heart 'blow', so you get stagnant columns of superficial blood. Varicose veins are not a contraindication for HRT. All HRT increases the risk of a deep vein thrombosis (DVT), which is a clot in the deep veins of your legs or pelvis. You can't take HRT if you have had a DVT or pulmonary embolus (PE). A PE is when the clot breaks off from a vein and travels into your lungs: these have a high risk of fatality. There is some evidence that HRT patches have a slightly lower risk of provoking clots than tablets, which is probably a dose effect. Obesity, increasing age, immobility, surgery, cancer, long-haul flights and smoking are all risk factors for a DVT.

I am on HRT. Are there any risks when I fly and should I be taking extra precautions?

There has been a lot in the press about the risk of venous thrombosis (blood clots in the veins) on long-haul flights and it is true that being on HRT may make the risk slightly higher. However, do not stop your HRT, but rather take sensible measures to reduce the risk. All passengers should carry out simple stretching exercises during the flight such as extension and flexion of the ankles to promote good circulation. You should drink plenty of water and consider the use of support socks that are available from chemists. If you have previously experienced a thrombosis, you should seek the advice of your doctor as to whether any other precautions are necessary.

Chapter 4

Will I put on weight with HRT? If so, which type of HRT will cause the least weight gain?

It is not inevitable that women gain weight on HRT, although some women do feel that it causes them to do so. Unfortunately, weight gain is common around the time that women usually start HRT (i.e. at mid-life), so it may feel as if the HRT is the cause, when in fact it is simply a lifestyle issue. Around mid-life, women often become more sedentary and, although they may not eat more, their bodies may actually need less to stay at the same weight – very unfair! Occasionally, women do experience a bloating feeling on HRT (contributing to no more than a pound or two in weight gain), which may be corrected by a change in dose or type of HRT. Changing from a cyclical to a continuous type of HRT may help women who are definitely through the menopause (i.e. no natural periods for at least one year). Using the lowest effective dose is also important as well as re-evaluating your food intake and exercise pattern. One product may suit you more than another, but there is no one HRT which is better for weight than another.

I am 45 and I suffer from migraines. Do they get worse at the menopause? Does HRT have any effect on migraines?

The great news is that at the menopause your migraines should get better, especially if you have the common sort of premenstrual migraine, just before a period. You may have a slightly stormy patch when your hormones are all over the place in the perimenopause, as your periods are petering out, but then you'll be liberated. I have seen just one case of a woman who only had migraines after the menopause; it is rare. As migraines are hormonally triggered, some women get terrible migraines on HRT, and this is a reason to stop treatment, just as if you got migraines on the contraceptive pill.

I have been taking oestrogen-only HRT for seven years. I am 57. I had a hysterectomy when I was 40 but still have my ovaries. I feel good on HRT and am concerned that if I come off it I will feel my general wellbeing deteriorate. Having read much conflicting information in both the medical (I am a radiographer) and popular press and hearing conflicting advice from various health professionals, I am unsure how to proceed. What advice can you give me?

Certainly it seems that oestrogen-only HRT is safer than combined oestrogen and progestogen from the breast cancer view-point.

I think the rational approach is to be on the lowest possible dose. Women need less oestrogen as they go though the menopause. At 57, I would expect you to be on 0.5 mg oestradiol or the equivalent. Speak to your doctor about lowering your dose. You can cut your tablets or patches in half, and keep on that dose for a few months, and then reduce it further. Only by weaning yourself off very slowly will you know if your wellbeing will really deteriorate, or not.

I am having hot flushes. I am thinking of starting HRT but I am worried about this and I hear that many women are apprehensive. What is your view about who can go on HRT?

The decision about whether or not to take HRT is complex. Oestrogen is the most effective treatment to relieve hot flushes and night sweats. It is important, however, that you have thought about how much these symptoms interfere with your life. This may provide the justification you are seeking if life has become a misery and you just cannot cope. Ask yourself what else is happening to you that is troublesome now or may become a future problem. If these problems would also be helped by hormones then it strengthens the case for taking HRT. If, however, the flushes are the only problem you have and are tolerable, but you have other health reasons that might make hormone therapy a risk, then it may not be the best choice. Deciding on HRT is an individual choice based on personal health analysis and a full understanding of the potential for benefits and risks that it may offer you specifically.

I have had chronic fatigue syndrome/ME for 20 years. I am 55 and very immobile. My energy levels in the past dipped severely when I had a period. I now have the menopause but still get severe dips of energy lasting up to several weeks. These could be hormonal, so I would like to try HRT. I don't want to get a stroke/heart attack. Am I at increased risk because of my immobility or would HRT give me more energy and make me more mobile, potentially counterbalancing the risks associated with taking it?

Taking some antidepressants, like fluoxetine, and doing planned exercise programmes can improve stamina in chronic fatigue patients. Immobility is a major risk factor for osteoporosis, so you need to ask your GP for a DXA bone scan, which will give information about what your bones are doing. You can then make an informed choice, as there are lots of treatments for osteoporosis, HRT being only one option. The risk of a stroke or heart attack at 55 is extremely small. However, there will be an extra risk of clots in your legs (a deep vein thrombosis, often called a DVT) possibly leading to a pulmonary embolism, (often called a PE) on HRT if you are that immobile. My patients with ME seem extra sensitive to any drugs, but you could try HRT at an extremely low dose, if you felt the benefits for you outweighed the risks. Discuss your risks for HRT with your doctor. It has to be your choice.

Over the last 12 months I have had blood tests, which have shown that I have some arthritis in the spine and back. My general health is good. My GP has suggested that I go back on HRT for a specified short time (two months) because it may eliminate my aches and pains which are my main problem. Having been on HRT for 12 years, come off it and suffered a very uncomfortable and painful year, I am somewhat reluctant to do this. My GP says that as I have only been off HRT for 15 months, it's safe to do this at present. Should the symptoms go, then I have to consider the merits or otherwise of remaining on HRT. But it occurs to me that if I follow this course, the discomforts clear up and I decide to stay on HRT, I will have to come off it again should a serious health problem arise in later years. In view of the above, I currently feel that I am going around in circles. Have you any advice to offer me? Would a blood test for polymyalgia be useful?

You don't actually specify which blood test you have had for arthritis. I'm afraid there are many different types. The commonest form of wear and tear arthritis is osteoarthritis, which we all have to some extent. This may be helped by chrondroitin and glucosamine supplements. Rheumatoid arthritis is an inflammatory auto-immune disease, which may lead to destruction of the joints and needs specialist supervision from a rheumatologist. There are then the group of 'sero-negative' arthritises (SLE, Reiter's, etc) which are even more difficult to treat. Then there are muscles diseases like polymyalgia, which are diagnosed and treated in general practice with high dose steroids. There is a group of women who come off HRT and get terrible aches and pains, without any change in blood test parameters. The aches wear off after a few months, but some of these women make an informed evidence-based choice to stay on HRT. It's up to you to decide about HRT. I think it would do no harm to talk all this over with your local rheumatologist.

At the age of 39 I had a hysterectomy and started taking HRT tablets. That was nearly five years ago. Could the HRT be responsible for my feelings of depression that I seem to be prone to now? My GP lowered my dose from 2 to 1 milligrams a day which seems to have helped a bit. For how long would you recommend that I continue taking HRT and then how should I come off of it when the time is right?

Let's start with the easy answer – you should continue HRT until 51, the age of the natural menopause. You have had an artificially early menopause because of the operation and you will be at considerable risk of osteoporosis without HRT. It is safe to take HRT under these circumstances as it is replacing the hormones that your body needs. When it is time to stop, you should prepare yourself by gradually cutting down on the dose of hormone and taking other measures to cope with hot flushes.

Your depression may not have anything to do with your HRT, as it is a common problem in the UK, especially in women. However, HRT can help lower the active testosterone in your body, which may add to feelings of lethargy. If you had your ovaries removed at the time of your hysterectomy you may be experiencing a lack of testosterone, since ovaries are an important source of testosterone. You could consider changing your HRT to tibolone (Livial) or adding a testosterone product to your existing medication. Depression usually responds well to a course of antidepressants and/or cognitive behavioural therapy. You should also have your thyroid hormone levels checked.

How much does HRT protect against osteoporosis?

Osteoporosis means the loss of bone mineral density to a level where the person has a higher risk of breaking a bone with very low trauma. Men and women start to lose bone density at the rate of 1 per cent a year from the age of 40 onwards, but women tend to lose bone density at a higher rate for around five years when they go through the menopause. This extra loss of bone density is due to the loss of oestrogen. By taking HRT, and therefore oestrogen, you get some benefit, with maintenance of your bone density. Some US research[8] has shown that if HRT is taken for up to five years, you reduce your risks for osteoporosis and fractures. The data from this research have recently been reanalysed and medical experts now suggest that most women will get more overall benefit than not if they take HRT between the ages of 50 and 60. However, with aging and the longer use of HRT, risks may start to outweigh benefits from the age of 60 . The benefit to your bones may not last once you stop HRT, but there are non-hormonal osteoporosis treatments that you could take if required.

For how long should HRT be taken to prevent osteoporosis?

How long you decide to take HRT for will depend on your own HRT risk-benefit evaluation, so this varies from woman to woman. This evaluation will decide whether you should take HRT or not, and needs to be repeated on a yearly basis. Whilst you are on HRT, this will help to reduce your loss of bone mineral density, as well as control your symptoms (including the typical hot flushes and night sweats). However, you need to discuss with your doctor certain risk factors, including those for breast cancer, strokes and thrombosis (blood clots in the legs). In general, current medical consensus is that the overall benefits of HRT may outweigh the risks for women between the ages of 50 and 60, but that with the long duration of HRT use and after the age of 60, the risks may start to outweigh the benefits of HRT. In the UK, the National Institute of Clinical Excellence (NICE) has suggested that bisphosphonates should be the first line of treatment for osteoporosis, and not HRT. Work by NICE is currently ongoing to look at the place of HRT for osteoporosis in comparison with all available bone sparing treatments.

Please can you give me the guidelines for going on HRT after a premature menopause, primary or secondary.

For how long should HRT be used?

The use of HRT is recommended to prevent complications of an early menopause, such as osteoporosis and fractures in later life. HRT can also help with the menopausal symptoms, which can be more severe after an early menopause.

HRT should be started as soon as the diagnosis has been made or immediately after the ovaries have been removed in a young woman. HRT usage should be reviewed around the age of 51 years, as this is the average age of the menopause in the UK. There is no reason to stop HRT after five years of use, as the benefits greatly outweigh the very low risks in those with an early menopause.

Chapter 5

Complementary therapies

Some women can't take HRT or don't want to. Other options are available, with many women choosing from a wide range of complementary therapies. Some therapies are backed by medical research, and may be recommended by some health professionals for menopausal symptoms.

When choosing a complementary therapy, it's wise to do some research first, looking at what it involves, where it's available and whether it's safe. Many therapies can be used alongside conventional treatments. But some therapies may not be safe for you, depending on your medical history (e.g. any medical conditions or any medication that you are on).

The most common therapies used at the menopause are acupuncture/acupressure, aromatherapy, herbal medicine, homeopathy, hypnotherapy, meditation, reflexology, relaxation, yoga and Tai chi. Choose a therapy that you are most comfortable with.

For the best effect, essential oils and herbal and homeopathic remedies can be tailor-made for the individual. So it's important to seek out a well-qualified, registered and regulated practitioner. Ideally, get a recommendation from someone you know or go through a reputable organisation.

Some remedies are available from pharmacies and health food stores with various claims. Check these out with a pharmacist or practitioner first to make sure they are suitable for your symptoms. If you decide to buy herbal or homeopathic products, buy them from a reputable supplier and make sure that they are manufactured by established companies that make good-quality products. You should learn how to use remedies properly before you take them, and always tell your doctor if you are using complementary therapies. Herbs in particular should be used with caution, as they can cause adverse effects and may interact with medicines you are taking. Some herbs may contain oestrogen-like substances that are not suitable for some women.

I am taking black cohosh. I've been taking it for six weeks and I've found no improvement. Should I be taking other herbal supplements as well such as red clover and agnus castus?

Many women use alternative therapies to treat hot flushes and other menopausal symptoms. Trials of black cohosh and other herbal treatments, such as agnus castus, provide conflicting results. It is still unclear whether these are any more effective than placebo (dummy treatment). Recently there have been reports of liver damage with black cohosh, so the current recommendation is that if you try black cohosh you should only do so for a maximum of six months. Black cohosh should also not be taken with blood pressure medications. Phytoestrogens, such as red clover, (oestrogens obtained from plant type sources) may be effective, with some reports that these help with the control of hot flushes. Phytoestrogens are sometimes thought of as replicating food sources of pulses (such as lentils or beans family) and therefore considered safer than medicines such as HRT as people think of these as more natural. But we know that herbal remedies are not safer. It's just that they have not been studied so extensively. Although phytoestrogens and black cohosh appear to be safe when used for short periods of time, much larger and longer studies are needed to understand whether long-term use is safe.

I am 66 years old. I came off HRT a year ago and I experienced menopausal symptoms. I started to take black cohosh drops six months ago. For how long can I take these safely? What other options do I have?

Black cohosh is a herb that is sometimes suggested to relieve menopausal symptoms. It is considered to be safe for most women, although there has not been much work on its long-term safety. There have been reports of liver damage following apparent use of black cohosh. It is thought that this is very rare, but short-term treatment of up to six months is usually suggested.

In the UK, herbal remedies are not yet licensed in the same way as conventional medicines. This means that there is no standardisation of dose or quality of product to rely on. If you have been recommended to try black cohosh by a health professional, it is worth checking the dose or type that they suggest.

Other options include isoflavones (such as red clover supplements) or complementary therapies like reflexology, aromatherapy or acupuncture. Complementary therapies may increase general wellbeing, even though they may not treat individual symptoms.

Medicines other than HRT (for example, clonidine and pro-gestogens) can be prescribed for menopausal symptoms. Eventually the symptoms should subside of their own accord.

I have heard that the herb sage can help women at the menopause. Is this true? If so, how should it be taken and what symptoms does it help?

Sage is a herb that can reduce menopausal hot flushes, exces-sive sweating and sore throats. It contains isoflavones, which are a type of phytoestrogen (plant oestrogen) that are also found in soya beans. Sage is mostly recommended to be taken as a tea, but the recipes vary. One option is to add two tea-spoons of dried sage to 250 ml boiling water, cover, steep and strain, then drink a cup at bedtime or during the day if neces-sary. Another option is to add three to five fresh sage leaves in a cup of hot, not boiling, water. The tea can be gargled to ease a sore throat. This herb is also used in cooking savory dishes, especially with pork.

When you are taking herbal remedies, I suggest you use one at a time for one to two weeks, starting in a tea form, with half a cup per day at first, increasing gradually. Monitor your symp-toms and stop if there are any side effects.

There are also sage tablets available to buy from health food shops. Remember that these tablets are classed as a food sup-plement rather than a medicine and have not had the stringent testing that all drugs go through. Sage acts as a weak oestrogen and may interfere with some prescribed medications and should be used with caution in some serious illnesses (e.g. breast can-cer), so check with your GP first.

How safe are herbal products for use during the menopause?

A lack of adequate clinical trials makes it difficult to comment on the overall risks or benefits of herbs. Women who decide to use alternative treatments, including herbs, should consult a registered practitioner. Some information is available about herbs used for specific reasons during the menopause. Phytoestrogens are currently fashionable, with small studies[9] showing benefit for symptoms such as hot flushes. Although they are generally considered to be safe treatments, their safety for long-term use or combined with HRT has not yet been assessed. Hot flushes may also be helped by St John's wort, black cohosh root extract and Dong quai. With some of these products, interactions with western medicines have been reported. Therefore, always check with your doctor or pharmacist first before you use them.

Hormone disturbances have been treated with herbs such as chaste tea, wild yam and false unicorn root. An Australian study[10] assessed the effects of a cream formulation containing wild yam extract on menopausal symptoms, cholesterol and sex hormones in 23 healthy menopausal women. It reported that short-term treatment is free from side effects, but appeared to have little effect on menopausal symptoms.

Other treatments that have been suggested include a bedtime drink of honey and hot water with three drops of sage essential oil to relieve night sweating. Regular drinks of camomile tea and lime blossom tea act as general relaxants. Passiflora tablets may help to reduce tension and anxiety, while oats act as a gentle tonic.

Can you give me information on the use of the herb Dong quai for menopausal symptoms?

Dong quai (*Angelica sinesisis*) is a herb that grows in China, Korea and Japan. Chinese practitioners use it as a nourishing blood tonic and to promote circulation. It is given to women to regulate the menstrual cycle, to balance female hormones, to calm nerves and to prevent troublesome symptoms of the menopause and premenstrual syndrome. The herb is a source of vitamins E, A and B12, iron and cobalt. You will need to consult a Chinese herbal practitioner for appropriate doses. Generally the herb is taken for eight to 12 weeks. Towards the end of the course, you should notice treatment effects. The costs will vary depending on where you obtain your supply.

Dong quai is just one of the commonly used herbal medicines for the menopause. However, there has been very little research into traditional medicines to show that it helps. Dong quai is not recommended during pregnancy, for women with excessive menstrual flow or for people taking blood thinning agents, so speak to your pharmacist first in these cases.

Is there evidence that natural progesterone cream helps menopausal symptoms or osteoporosis? Is it safe?

Some women who have used natural progesterone cream feel that it helps to control their menopausal symptoms. So far, however, there's little research, and no convincing studies have shown any improvement in menopausal symptoms or osteoporosis. The question of whether it is safe is also controversial. Again, there is not enough research evidence. You should be aware that when you see a doctor for HRT, following a risk-benefit evaluation, you will be prescribed oestrogen. Progestogen will be added to protect you from endometrial hyperplasia (a non-cancerous condition where the womb lining builds up more than usual) and cancer if you still have a uterus (i.e. no hysterectomy). Whether natural progesterone cream also provides effective endometrial (womb lining) protection is really not known. The other question is whether progestogens increase or decrease the risk of breast cancer. Again, we don't know the answer to this as yet. If your GP gives you a prescription for natural progesterone cream, this will have to be a private prescription. The reason why your GP can't prescribe natural progesterone cream on the NHS is because the related research is very weak. Many women say they can buy supplies over the internet, but I would not recommend this, as you may be putting yourself at risk. It is always good to get professional advice, so you may wish to check with your GP.

I have read that evening primrose oil can help hot flushes. Is this true and has there been any research on it?

Two reviews, one from a US research team in February 2006[11] and one from a Scandanavian group in October 2005[12], looked at the research behind various treatments to help control menopausal symptoms such as hot flushes. Both suggest that the evidence to support the use of evening primrose oil for hot flushes is very weak. The recommendation is that further research be carried out to help answer the question on whether some of these treatments, including evening primrose oil, can be advocated as a treatment for menopause symptom control.

Which homeopathic remedies help menopausal symptoms?

Homeopathy aims to kick-start a woman's own body into healing itself and it aims to cure 'like with like'. Few studies have evaluated its effectiveness at the time of the menopause, but some small studies have shown an early indication of benefit on hot flushes and mood swings. Homeopathic treatment should be on an individual basis administered by a qualified homeopath or homeopathic doctor. Treatments which might be tailored for use include Sepia, Pulsatilla, *Lachesis mutus* (for hot flushes), Valerian (for sweating), *Ferrum metallicum* (for hot flushes and exhaustion), Sulphur (for night sweats) and *Lycopodium clavatum* (for vaginal dryness). More studies are needed before homeopathy can be recommended.

Chapter 6
Nutrition

Members of The Menopause Exchange send in questions on various aspects of nutrition, so this chapter is divided into three sections: general nutrition, phytoestrogens, and vitamins and minerals. These relate to healthy eating, dietary supplements, the menopause and osteoporosis.

Small dietary changes can help to ease many menopausal symptoms, reduce the risk of chronic diseases (including heart disease), strengthen bones and control weight. Although it's better to obtain nutrients from your diet, some women do turn to dietary supplements. When buying supplements, read the instructions first. Bear in mind that they can affect any medication that you are taking and that some shouldn't be taken if certain medical conditions are present. Check with a pharmacist or other health professional before buying them.

There is much interest in the role of phytoestrogens in easing menopausal symptoms. Phytoestrogens are a group of plant hormones that have a chemical structure similar to the body's natural oestrogen, but they are hundreds of thousands of times weaker than oestrogen. They include some foods and herbs that affect hormonal balance. Some women find phytoestrogens helpful for reducing both the frequency and severity of hot flushes. There are two main dietary types of phytoestrogens: isoflavones and lignans. Isoflavones are found in soya bean products, like tofu and soya milk, beans, pulses and chick peas. Lignans are found in fibre-rich foods, including some fruit and vegetables, wheatbran and seeds such as linseed.

Calcium has a major part to play in maintaining bone health, as it strengthens the collagen framework of bones. Calcium absorption decreases with age. You also need vitamin D to ensure that calcium is properly absorbed into your body. Other vitamins and minerals, such as magnesium, selenium and iron, are also important for good health.

There are two basic groups of vitamins: fat-soluble ones and water-soluble ones. The water-soluble vitamins include the B group and vitamin C. These are needed every day, as your body can't store them. Fat-soluble vitamins, which include vitamins A, D and E, can be stored by your body in small amounts, so they are not needed absolutely every day.

***

General nutrition

Please can you give me some tips on eating healthily at the menopause?

Your passage through the menopause may be easier if you eat a healthy balanced diet. Maintaining a healthy weight means fewer hot flushes and a lower risk of developing certain cancers and heart disease, so watch the amount of fat you eat, especially saturated fats (mainly animal origin). Try to have one to two portions of oily fish a week to benefit your heart and joints and as a source of bone-protecting vitamin D. Plant oestrogens (phytoeostrogens), e.g. soya milk, may help with hot flushes and protect against some cancers. Remember to take in enough bone-building calcium, in milk products, beans and green vegetables. Finally, don't forget to have at least five portions of fruit and/or vegetables a day to keep cancer and heart disease at bay.

Does diet affect the menopause, for example eating a lot of chocolate, crisps and nuts? Are there any other foods that might trigger menopausal symptoms or make them worse?

The key to a manageable menopause is to start with a healthy balanced diet in order to avoid exacerbating symptoms. Aim for three meals a day (plus healthy snacks if needed) based on wholegrain carbohydrates, plenty of fruit and vegetables (which are rich in antioxidants), low fat dairy products (for a boost to calcium intake), and lean meats and fish for iron and protein. While occasional treats are fine, lots of sugary and fatty snacks such as chocolate and crisps are likely to promote weight gain and increase the risk of heart disease. Hot flushes can be made worse by hot foods and drinks, spicy foods, caffeine and alcohol, so it's worth checking if these affect you. Eating foods rich in phytoestrogens every day, such as soya products, can help to reduce hot flushes. And don't forget regular moderate activity to help with mood swings and weight control and to prevent osteoporosis and heart disease.

I have read that I should be eating five portions a day of fruit and vegetables for good health. Which are best: fresh, frozen, tinned or dried fruits and vegetables?

The five-a-day message applies to all forms of fruit and vegetables, including fruit or vegetable juices or smoothies. It is best to have a good variety, so you shouldn't have all of your five a day as juice or canned products or as one type of vegetable or fruit. Nutritionists also recommend that you try to have a mixture of colours from fruits and vegetables, as you will then ensure that you eat a variety of antioxidants.

As a simple rule, I would recommend at least three of your five portions come from fresh or frozen fruit and vegetables, and then have the other two as other forms. If they are not stored for too long in the freezer, frozen vegetables retain most of their nutritional value and so are as good as fresh. The five-a-day message is really a minimum target so feel free to have more than this!

My GP has told me that my cholesterol levels are a little high, but not high enough to warrant medication. Can you suggest dietary ways of lowering my cholesterol levels? Which foods should I avoid and which should I eat more of?

The best way of reducing high cholesterol is to check your weight, and if you are overweight to reduce it by following a balanced, but calorie-reduced diet.

In addition, and if you have no weight to lose, you should try to follow a diet that is not too high in fatty foods. Furthermore, the fats you do eat should be unsaturated rather than saturated fats, as these tend to raise cholesterol levels. Saturated fats are found in fatty meat, sausages, pies and pastry (unless made with unsaturated fat), whole milk, cream, butter and lard.

Unsaturated fats are found in nuts and seeds (plus oils extracted from them), sunflower, olive and rapeseed (groundnut) oils, sunflower or olive oil based margarines. Look for those that claim to help reduce cholesterol.

Eating a diet high in soluble fibre may also help to bring down cholesterol levels; this includes fruit, vegetables, oats and pulses.

I have read about probiotic yoghurt drinks and supplements. Will a daily yoghurt drink or a supplement benefit me and in what way?

The gut is full of bacteria which aid digestion and help to fight off tummy bugs. The balance between friendly and unfriendly bacteria in your gut influences general health for both adults and children. The friendly bacteria live off certain types of carbohydrate called prebiotics, which are found in low levels in bananas, chicory, asparagus and leeks. If you are having a healthy high fibre diet with lots of fruit and vegetables you may be eating sufficient prebiotics to maintain lots of friendly gut bacteria. However, if you eat a low fibre diet, you may be out of balance and drinking or eating a probiotic may boost the levels of friendly bacteria. Bear in mind that these will only top up your bacteria levels and do not provide the food they need to survive. If you take these, eating a healthier diet will help too. In addition, having a probiotic food or drink can help get your gut back in balance following a stomach bug or course of antibiotics.

What effect does drinking too much alcohol have on the menopause and on bones?

Alcohol drunk to excess can lead to a loss of bone mass at any age. The menopause itself causes an accelerated loss of bone mass. You don't want to be exacerbating this by drinking too much. For women, the maximum level of alcohol taken a week should be 14 units. Remember this no longer equates to a pub-measure glass of wine or even half a pint of beer/larger or cider due to the larger glass size of wine now served and the strength of many alcoholic drinks having risen.

Alcohol can also exacerbate hot flushes, along with anxiety and depression during the menopause. And don't forget that alcoholic drinks are pretty calorie-loaded, so they make it even harder to avoid midlife weight gain.

I have read that some drinks are bad for the bones. Is this true? If so, which drinks have this effect and why?

There are three types of drinks that can affect bone health:
Alcohol: this is a definite risk factor if drunk to excess, as alcohol hinders the bone-forming cells. However, it has been shown that sensible intakes of one or two glasses of red wine per day may actually protect the skeleton.
Caffeine: the effect is not great, but if you have other risk factors it may be worth limiting your intake. The main evidence[13] has been for black coffee, whereas tea appears to not have an effect and may even be protective. Excess coffee is believed to cause increased calcium loss in the urine.
Fizzy drinks: phosphoric acid is used as a preservative in some canned fizzy drinks. Excess consumption of these drinks may cause calcium to be leached from the bones. However, the evidence for this is still not very strong.

Can you advise what I can do to help me to stop craving food every afternoon? I am going through the perimenopause.

If you are genuinely hungry, then you need to make sure you have had enough to eat at lunch time. If you are trying to cut down on food intake too much at lunch times, it may leave you feeling so hungry later that you succumb to nibbling all afternoon. Also make sure that your lunch provides you with food that will keep you feeling full for a long time afterwards; some lean protein and starchy wholegrain foods are good for this. There is nothing wrong with having a nutritious snack in the afternoon, especially if you have a long gap between your lunch and evening meal. A handful of dried fruit and unsalted nuts is ideal for staving off hunger.

Sometimes boredom, lack of activity, tiredness or thirst can trigger a desire to eat, so make sure you are not wrongly assuming that what you need is food!

I have read that garlic is good for you, especially in warding off colds and flu and boosting your circulation. Is this true? Should I eat more garlic or can I take supplements to get any benefits?

There is some evidence[14, 15] that garlic, and garlic extract found in supplements, may have anti-clotting and anti-oxidant properties and so may help keep cancer and heart disease at bay. However, the scientific trials have been done on animals and cell lines and this is not hard evidence that it works equally well in whole humans! There is growing evidence from some studies in humans that garlic has cholesterol- and blood pressure-lowering effects, reduces inflammation and can help ward off colds. However, before you get too excited, there is still not enough evidence to make garlic the new wonder drug! There is no real harm in taking garlic, although it can irritate the stomach.

Phytoestrogens

Please can you tell me about the use of phytoestrogens at the menopause. Do they have any side effects?

Phytoestrogens are also known as plant oestrogens, due to their similarity in chemical structure to oestrogen. Eating foods rich in phytoestrogens, such as soya, soya foods and linseeds, can help to reduce the number and severity of hot flushes during the menopause, and may also help protect against osteoporosis and heart disease. To reduce menopausal symptoms, it is thought that intakes need to be around 40 to 80 milligrams of phytoestrogens per day, which would be found in a serving of textured vegetable protein, tofu or soya beans plus a glass of soya milk daily.

Are there any medical conditions that could stop women being able to take phytoestrogens (a substantial amount in food or phytoestrogen supplements)? Can phytoestrogens affect any medication that is being taken?

Phytoestrogens are safe for most women. However, if you are taking thyroxine, for an underactive thyroid, phytoestrogens may interfere with the drug's effectiveness. This doesn't mean you need to avoid phytoestrogens, but if you are consciously increasing the amount you eat (for example, to help with hot flushes), ask your GP to monitor your thyroxine levels and adjust the dose accordingly. The only other group who should be cautious of phytoeestrogens is women at a high risk of developing breast cancer or who have oestrogen-dependent breast cancer. At the moment, it is not clear whether phytoestrogens affect the risk of the development or growth of breast cancer, but until the research evidence is available, it is probably better to be cautious and avoid eating large amounts of phytoestrogens or taking phytoestrogen supplements.

Which foods contain phytoestrogens? How much phytoestrogen do these foods contain and how much phytoestrogen should women going through the menopause take in each day?

The main type of phytoestrogens in the diet are isoflavones. They act like a weak oestrogen during and after the menopause. A total of 50 milligrams isoflavone per day is believed to be required to help relieve some menopausal symptoms, including hot flushes. It may take up to 12 weeks to start seeing any beneficial effects, and taking a fish oil supplement with the phytoestrogen may enhance its effect. Although several seeds, nuts, fruits, vegetables and beans are sources of phytoestrogens, soya is the richest source.

Product	Isoflavone per 100 gram	Serving size	Isoflavone per serving
Soya milk	10 milligrams	250 millilitres	26 milligrams
Soya yogurt	10 milligrams	125 grams	13 milligrams
Textured vegetable protein (soya mince)	33 milligrams	75 grams	25 milligrams

What dose of phytoestrogen should I be taking in a supplement? For how long can I take phytoestrogen supplements?

Phytoestrogens (usually isoflavones) are sometimes suggested to help ease menopausal symptoms. The evidence backing their use is mixed, and it is unclear which dose might be most effective. In studies, doses used have varied from 30 to 140 milligrams,[9] occasionally even more. Although large doses are used in studies, in practice no more than about 80 milligrams should be taken a day. Taking one 40 milligram tablet a day of a product containing isoflavones might be effective for menopausal symptoms, increasing to one tablet twice a day if necessary.

Another complication is that there are many different products available, but not all are clear as to how much of the phytoestrogen they contain. As to how long you can take them, it is assumed that phytoestrogens are safe to use in the long term but there are no studies supporting this. Women with breast cancer should use isoflavones with caution.

Is it better to increase the amount of phytoestrogens in my diet or to take phytoestrogen supplements?

We assume that it is better to increase phytoestrogens in your diet, as phytoestrogen-rich foods tend to be low in fat and high in fibre, which carries other health benefits. Good sources of dietary phytoestrogens include linseeds, tofu or soya products, as well as alfalfa, cherries, garlic and lentils. Women on special diets or who don't like these foods may prefer taking a tablet. There are different types of phytoestrogens, so choose a brand containing all four for maximum benefit. Some supplements are pricey, so check carefully and look out for introductory offers, making sure that they contain what you require.

I am on HRT. Can I also increase the amount of phytoestrogens in my diet or take phytoestrogen supplements?

Phytoestrogens have a much weaker hormonal effect compared with HRT and hopefully the HRT is taking care of most of your menopausal symptoms. However, it is thought that the body uses different types of oestrogen in slightly different ways, so increasing your intake of phytoestrogen-rich foods while taking HRT may still have benefits. The foods rich in phytoestrogens are also great sources of soya protein and soluble fibre, which are known to help look after the heart. Eating these rather than taking supplements will give you added value. Foods rich in phytoestrogens include soya beans and soya foods such as milks, yoghurts, TVP (textured vegetable protein) and other soya meat substitutes, linseed and rye. Try to eat a serving of one of these foods a couple of times every day.

I'm becoming increasingly worried by the number of women who embark on special menopause diets and then feed the whole family on these foods. I have read that male and female dietary requirements are quite different and that there is concern that the high levels of soya in processed foods 'feminises' men. Aren't women on high soya diets risking the health of their male family members?

In short, no. There is no need to fear putting the males of the household at risk by increasing the amount of soya, and as a result phytoestrogens, in their diets. A review by the UK Committee on Toxicology of Chemicals in Food, Consumer Products and the Environment, Phytoestrogens and Health, published in 2003[16] found no links between the intake of soya foods, phytoestrogens (from foods or supplements) and male sex hormone levels or sperm count. In fact, the protein in soya and soluble fibre that the beans contain are both known to help to maintain a healthy heart, so eating more soya foods is likely to be of benefit to the general health of all the family.

Vitamins and minerals

All my friends are taking food supplements – antioxidants, garlic, fish oils, for example. Now that I am getting older, should I be taking supplements too or is eating a balanced diet enough for good health?

A healthy balanced diet should provide all the nutrition that you need. However, we live hectic lives and don't always manage to eat an ideal diet every day. Supplements complement a healthy diet, but should never be used instead of healthy eating. Taking a cocktail of supplements can mean too much of a good thing. For example, multivitamins and cod liver oil contain vitamins A and D; taking both will mean a high intake which could be harmful.

The golden rules for supplements are:

- Be aware – don't double up or take more than recommended.
- Buy a reputable brand – they cost a bit more but are more

likely to contain what they say on the label.
- Check out claims – just because the manufacturer says it will work doesn't mean that it is true.
- Check with a pharmacist about interactions between vitamins, minerals, herbal supplements and prescription medications, as these are common.

I am 63 and in good health and I am not taking any medication. What are the most important vitamins and minerals that I should look out for at my age and which foods contain them? If I can't or don't eat the foods that you suggest, would food supplements help and, if so, which ones should I take?

There is little change in the recommended intakes of vitamins and minerals with age, apart from vitamin D. There is no recommended intake for vitamin D in the under-65s, as this vitamin is made in the skin from sunlight, but the recommended intake is 10 micrograms per day in the over-65s. This is mainly to do with the reduced exposure of the skin to sunlight as we get older, rather than a change in our ability to produce the vitamin. Some foods should feature regularly in your diet. Oily fish (e.g. salmon or mackerel) provide omega-3s to protect your heart and vitamin D for your bones, while dairy foods boost your calcium intake. Fortified breakfast cereals provide iron, vitamin D and B vitamins, while colourful fruit and vegetables provide protective antioxidants. If you want to take a supplement, choose a one-a-day multivitamin and mineral with an omega-3 supplement if desired.

How much calcium do women, going through the menopause, need each day? Is this amount the same for women after the menopause and at different ages?

You are right to be thinking about your calcium intake as the menopause is an important time for bone health, and a good calcium intake may help the loss of calcium from the bones. The dietary reference value for adults is 700 milligrams per day. The National Osteoporosis Society recommends an intake of 1200 milligrams calcium per day for those who have been diagnosed with osteoporosis.

The richest sources of calcium in the diet are dairy foods. One third of a pint of semi-skimmed milk provides 231 milligrams, a carton of yoghurt 190 milligrams, and 28 grams (one ounce) of cheese 200 milligrams. Other good sources include canned fish, such as pilchards (300 milligrams/100 grams) or sardines (460 milligrams/100 grams), kale, watercress or spinach (150 milligrams/100 grams) and tofu (510 milligrams/100 grams). Other things you can do to help with bone health are to take regular weight-bearing exercise, quit smoking and moderate alcohol intake.

More information on calcium and bone health can be obtained from the National Osteoporosis Society.

I have osteoarthritis, an overactive thyroid and an irregular heart beat. It is two and a half years since my last period. I have a 'healthy' diet and I eat fresh fruit and vegetables, natural yoghurt and cream cheese for calcium naturally. I have read that during the menopause I should take a calcium supplement and vitamins for the

'over 50s'. My nails are covered in white marks and a friend said this indicates a calcium deficiency. Should I take a calcium supplement and also vitamins? Do white marks mean calcium deficiency? As I have the above medical conditions, could extra vitamin supplements be a risk?

White flecks on your nails don't mean calcium deficiency, and for the most part happen when nails are damaged, primarily when they are still developing underneath and behind your cuticle. If you are not having three portions of low fat calcium rich foods a day (yoghurts, milk and hard cheese or alternatives such as fortified soya products), then a supplement is recommended, especially if you have been diagnosed with a low bone mass.

In order to absorb enough calcium, you need to have an adequate vitamin D status. This can be achieved by exposing yourself to some sunlight most days during the summer months. Oily fish, eggs, offal and spreads are a good dietary source too. (Spreads are what used to be known as margarines but because over 90 per cent of those on the market are lower in fat than they used to be, they cannot be relabelled as margarines and so are called fat spreads.) You may need to take a supplement if you don't go out much during daylight hours and don't eat these foods.

To conclude, you only need to take a supplement if your diet is inadequate or if your doctor has advised you to. If you are on any medication for other conditions, you should always check with your doctor before taking supplements or herbals.

I am 58. I know that I need vitamin D with calcium to help my bones and that sunlight is a source of vitamin D. How do I make sure that I get adequate supplies of vitamin D in the winter? Which foods are rich in vitamin D? Should I take a supplement?

Foods rich in vitamin D include oily fish, eggs, butter, margarine, fat spreads and fortified breakfast cereals. (Most fat spreads are fortified with vitamin D.) There is no UK recommended intake for vitamin D for women up to the age of 65, as it assumed that enough of the vitamin will be made by the body through the action of sunlight on the skin. So an adequate vitamin D status relies on you having allowed your skin to be exposed to sunlight during the summer. Some experts now believe that concerns over skin cancer are leading us to store insufficient vitamin D in the summer to see us through the winter. If you feel that you have not had enough sunlight exposure during the summer, then you may need a supplement of 10 micrograms of vitamin D a day.

Do I need to take magnesium in my diet in addition to calcium and vitamin D to help my bones? If so, which foods contain magnesium? Are there any other vitamins and minerals that I should be including for bone protection?

There is some evidence[17] that a significant percentage of women going through the menopause are deficient in magnesium; however, the jury is still out on how important magnesium is in bone health. To be on the safe side, make sure you have sufficient magnesium in the diet, which is found in wholegrains, green vegetables, beans, peas, nuts and seeds.

Calcium and vitamin D are the nutrients to pay most attention to regarding bone health, but evidence is gathering for the importance of antioxidants in the diet and for bone health. Isoflavones from foods such as soya products have been shown to have a protective effect on bone in animal studies. Evidence in humans, however, is conflicting.

Ensure you eat plenty of fruit and vegetables of all different colours for good health.

I have read that selenium is good for people as they age. Is this true? If so, what foods contain the most selenium? Are there selenium supplements?

Selenium has aroused great interest as a result of its antioxidant effects and therefore possible protective role against many diseases associated with ageing, such as heart disease. However, like all vitamins and minerals, taking in more selenium than the body needs will not lead to extra benefits. It is advisable not to exceed the recommended intake (60 micrograms a day for women).

Selenium is found in meat (especially liver), fish, cheese, nuts (particularly brazil nuts), bread, cereals (especially wholegrain) and lentils. If your diet is unbalanced, selenium intake may be low. This is particularly the case in the UK because the soil on which cereals are grown is selenium-deficient. Even so, if your diet is balanced and contains a regular amount of these selenium-rich foods, you should not need to take a supplement.

I am 51. What are the benefits of iron in the diet and in which foods is it present? How much iron should I be taking each day?

A shortage of iron is not normally a problem after the menopause. This is because the monthly bleed no longer happens, and this is what can be a big drain on a woman's iron reserves. Taking in too much iron can be harmful, so I certainly would not recommend taking supplements unless you have been diagnosed with iron deficiency anaemia by a doctor. From the age of 50 onwards, the recommended daily iron intake is 8.7 milligrams. (compared with 14.8 milligrams for 19-50 year olds). Red meat, liver and sardines are good sources, as are fortified breakfast cereals, beans, pulses and dried fruit.

Which antioxidants will help me at the time of the menopause? In which foods are they found? Should I be taking antioxidant supplements?

You need a whole spectrum of antioxidants right through life. For a start, you can get a wide range by eating at least five helpings a day of fruit and vegetables. Eating a variety of colours ensures a variety of antioxidants. Even chocolate (good quality and dark is best) and wine contain antioxidants. The antioxidant vitamins are vitamin E, vitamin C and the beta-carotene form of vitamin A. Minerals such as selenium, copper, manganese and zinc are combined with certain enzymes to provide antioxidant action. It is not just vitamins and minerals that act as antioxidants, but other substances found in fruit and vegetables (e.g. bioflavonoids) and fish, nuts and lean meats (e.g. co-enzyme Q^{10}) do too.

In general, antioxidants are believed to help protect against cancers and heart disease. However, recent research[18] has shown that isolating anti-oxidants and giving them to people in supplement form doesn't have the desired effect. In fact, in some cases the reverse tends to happen, with supplements being more likely to bring on the disease they are meant to prevent, such as heart disease with vitamins E supplements and a form of lung cancer in smokers who take beta-carotene supplements. My advice is stick to a good diet and lay off the antioxidant supplements.

Full fat dairy products are a good source of vitamin A but these are bad for cholesterol. What is your view on this?

Vitamin A is a fat-soluble vitamin and found only in foods containing fat. When the fat is removed from milk, the vitamin A is removed with it, hence the reference to full-fat milk and dairy foods. You are right that advice to lower cholesterol generally limits the intake of full fat dairy foods due to their saturated fat content. However there are alternative sources of vitamin A in a cholesterol-lowering diet, such as oily fish and polyunsaturated or monounsaturated spreads. A national dietary survey[19] showed that meat, meat products and vegetables are the biggest sources of vitamin A in the UK, and that dairy foods provide just 14 per cent of intake. In fact, reduced-fat milk made a bigger contribution than full-fat milk due to the larger amounts being consumed. In short, limiting full-fat dairy foods is unlikely to be harming your vitamin A intake.

I have read that we need to exercise care when taking vitamins with cod liver oil. I have been taking a multivitamin tablet with a 1000 milligram cod liver oil for years as well as other supplements. I haven't heard of this warning before. Am I lucky to be alive??!!

Vitamin A, if taken in excess, can be damaging to the liver. Most vitamin supplements contain 100 per cent (800 micrograms) or more of recommended intakes. Cod liver oil supplements (either capsules or liquid) also generally contain 800 micrograms vitamin A, or 100 per cent of vitamin A requirement in each capsule or dose. Therefore if you take both this and cod liver oil it is quite easy to find you are consuming double the amount of vitamin A that you actually need. In addition there is the vitamin A coming from the foods and drinks that you consume. Average daily intakes of vitamin A from food by UK women are 112 per cent of the recommended intake,[19] and so in theory we do not need to take additional vitamin A at all. Add together diet, multivitamin and cod liver oil and you are having at least three times your recommended intake of vitamin A. While there are some safety factors built into recommended intakes it is not advisable grossly to exceed these on a regular basis. If you wish to continue taking both a multivitamin and cod liver oil it is wise to check dosage, and an alternative may be to choose a pregnancy multivitamin as these do not contain any vitamin A.

I am 55 years old. I took HRT from the age of 45 to 53. (I had the whole of one ovary and part of the other removed surgically at the age of 42.) By the time I stopped taking HRT nearly three years ago, I seemed to have bypassed any symptoms I might have suffered and I have

felt fine, except for the odd twinge in the joints. I took cod liver oil capsules to keep my bones strong but I am worried that I shouldn't be taking cod liver oil on a regular basis at the menopause. Is this so, and would it also apply to other fish oils? I am not taking anything other than soya, linseed, pumpkin seeds etc. I would like to do whatever I can to help combat the onset of osteoporosis and to keep my bones and joints in as good a condition as possible. What advice can you give me?

The omega-3 oils found in oily fish and fish oil supplements may help with rheumatoid arthritis, which involves the body's immune system and inflammation of the joints. They are less likely to help with osteoarthritis, which is the most common form in older people and involves the cartilage in the joints becoming worn and ineffective. The best way to prevent osteoarthritis is to keep a healthy weight to reduce the strain on the joints and remain active. Fish oils will not help to prevent osteoporosis. The best approach for this is to ensure a good intake of calcium-rich foods in the diet (or take a reputable calcium supplement) and undertake weight-bearing activity (such as walking or dancing) on most days.

Taking more than an average of 1.5 milligrams of vitamin A daily over many years may increase the risk of bone fracture and osteoporosis. This amount is two and a half times the recommended intake of 600 micrograms per day for adult women. Fish liver oil supplements (as well as many multivitamins) are high in vitamin A. So if you take supplements containing vitamin A, make sure you don't have more than a total of 1.5 milligrams per day from your food and supplements. If you eat liver or liver products such as pâté every week, you should avoid taking any supplements that contain vitamin A, because liver is very rich in vitamin A. The best approach is to try to eat one to two servings of an oily fish each week (mackerel, pilchards, salmon, trout etc) or if you want to take a supplement choose an omega-3 rich fish oil supplement (which has the vitamin A removed) instead of cod liver oil.

Is vitamin E good for hot flushes and can everyone take vitamin E supplements?

Vitamin E has been noted[20] to cause a slightly greater reduction in hot flushes than dummy pills, but not as much as the oestrogens in HRT. Interestingly, it has been found that dummy pills on their own consistently reduce the number and severity of hot flushes by about 25 to 30 per cent. Vitamin E is usually well tolerated, although large doses may cause diarrhoea, abdominal pain and other digestive upsets. Large doses may increase the tendency to bleed in women with a deficiency in vitamin K (for example, those taking oral anti-coagulants).

I am going through the menopause. My nails have become brittle and my hair has become thinner. What vitamins and minerals would improve this and in which foods are they found? Please can you suggest any supplements that may help.

You can buy supplements that are said to benefit both nails and hair, but the best thing you can do for skin, nails and hair is to make sure you have a balanced diet, get plenty of sleep, take regular exercise and try to reduce stress levels in your life. Sometimes changes happen during the menopause, which no amount of supplementation can put right as they are due to the fall in oestrogen levels. If you have other menopausal symptoms you may wish to try a phytoestrogen (plant oestrogen) supplement, which may help to reverse some of the symptoms associated with the fall in oestrogen levels.

I have been told by my GP that my folic acid level is low. What causes this? Are there any foods that I should be eating to increase the level? Will I need to take a supplement?

Vitamin B^9 is the name given to natural folate (from the Latin word *folium*) and folic acid, an artificially produced form of the vitamin that is used as a supplement and to fortify foods. Your doctor will have measured your red blood cell folate level to determine if you are deficient or not. Deficiency gives rise to a form of anaemia and can be for a number of reasons, including having other disease states, such as kidney and liver disease or alcoholism, but a common reason is due to a diet low in this vitamin. For two to three months, take a 400 microgram supplement to improve your folic acid status, and ensure you eat a diet with plenty of green leafy vegetables, citrus fruits, some nuts and seeds, dried beans and peas. Fortified foods, such as fat spreads, yeast extract and breakfast cereals, are useful sources too. (Almost all fat spreads are now fortified with folic acid.)

Chapter 7

A Mixture of Options for Coping with the Menopause

Many women ask how they should cope with menopausal symptoms. Sometimes, the answers are not always clear-cut and they include a variety of approaches. This is why I have included this chapter.

Most of the questions in this chapter relate to hot flushes and night sweats. Methods of coping can include self-help measures and lifestyle changes. Self-help measures may be related to how you dress or how you sleep or other ways of cooling yourself down (e.g. using the cooling menthol effect of little film-like mint breath fresheners). Lifestyle changes may include increasing the amount of exercise that you do, avoiding anxiety-provoking situations and warm, stuffy rooms and making time for something that you enjoy. There are also prescription medicine alternatives to HRT, complementary therapies and nutrition.

Each expert will have their own ideas on how a particular woman should cope. Every woman is individual, depending on her symptoms, medical history and family medical history, so the advice given in this chapter won't be suitable for everyone.

***

I don't want to go on HRT. When I saw my doctor recently about my hot flushes, he suggested that I try a prescription drug alternative. Which of these work the best and do they have any side effects?

Non-oestrogen-based treatments may be considered for women who don't wish to take oestrogen-based HRT or who have a medical reason why they shouldn't take it. Most of these alternatives are not as good at relieving hot flushes as oestrogen. Low-dose progestogens (the other main female hormone) can be helpful. Clonidine (a drug prescribed for migraine or high blood pressure) is another option, but the usual dose of 50 to 75 micrograms is of limited benefit and has side effects, including sleeping difficulties, a dry mouth, dizziness, constipation and sedation. The antidepressants, selective serotonin re-uptake inhibitors (SSRIs) and serotonin norepinephrine re-uptake inhibitors (SNRIs), include fluoxetine, citalopram, paroxetine and venlafaxine. They are effective in treating hot flushes by up to 60 per cent in the short term. Venlafaxine also improves libido and mood. The dose has to be started low and gradually increased to minimise side effects (e.g. nausea, dizziness and sleep disturbance). Gabapentin can also be effective, reducing hot flushes by 40 to 50 per cent, especially in women experiencing aches and pains. This drug is used to treat epilepsy, migraine and nerve-related pain; again start on a low dose and increase slowly. Tiredness is the main side effect.

I prefer not to go on HRT and I have heard that a drug called venlafaxine can help hot flushes. Can you tell me about it?

Venlafaxine belongs to the SNRI (serotonin norepinephrine re-uptake inhibitors) class of antidepressants. Serotonin is a brain neurotransmitter, which jumps across gaps between nerve cells in the brain to take messages along pathways. Venlafaxine significantly reduces hot flushes in menopausal women when used in low doses. Women who have breast cancer can safely take it for hot flushes, as can other women who choose not to use HRT. It is best to start with a low dose at night-time.

(Editor's note: The use of the low dose (37.5 milligrams/day) of venlafaxine for hot flushes is half the initial dose used to treat depression and is associated with minimal side effects.)

My friend is taking clonidine and she has found that it has helped her hot flushes and night sweats. What is your opinion on it and can anyone take it?

Clonidine may help hot flushes but does not do so reliably and it is impossible to predict who will respond successfully. It was originally developed for the treatment of high blood pressure but it is rarely used even in this condition because of its range of adverse effects. These include dry mouth, sedation, depression, fluid retention, headaches and sleep disturbance. It therefore has the potential to create more problems than it solves. I only prescribe it occasionally when there are no more effective or safer options for the patient involved.

I am having a period every five to six months. How long does it have to be after my last period before I know that I have been through the menopause? What advice can

you give me for coping with the menopause when it arrives?

Once you have not seen a period for at least a year, this usually means you are in the menopause. At this time, you should be looking after your health, by eating a healthy diet, not smoking and exercising regularly. All these are general health measures, but the menopause may be time to double-check you are doing it right.

You should consider your bones. Are you at an increased risk of osteoporosis? Seek advice if you have already broken a bone, if your mother had a hip fracture or if you have regularly used corticosteroids. The menopause simply marks the end of your periods. If you do experience symptoms, don't be afraid to seek help.

I am 50 and having irregular periods. I am in good health and I don't seem to be experiencing any menopausal symptoms. What advice can you give me for looking after myself well during the perimenopause?

During the perimenopause, a health lifestyle and positive outlook on life bring many benefits. See your doctor or nurse for a blood pressure and cholesterol check, and go for your cervical smear test and mammogram when the invitation arrives. If your period become very heavy or you notice any bleeding in between the periods or after sex, report this to your GP. Don't forget to devote quality time to your partner and yourself and remember to use effective contraception until one year after your last natural period.

I have recently started waking up in the night feeling very hot, especially my hands and feet. I am not actually sweating but I have to throw the bedclothes off to cool down. This is happening at least twice a night. I am 51. Can you confirm if this is a sign of the menopause? I don't feel in control of my body at the moment and it is a bit scary. Do you have any tips or can you point me in the right direction?

It is indeed possible that the feelings of heat you are experiencing are due to changes in hormones leading up to the time of menopause. This is described as the perimenopause and can start before you see any changes to your periods. You can prepare a little for it by using cotton types of bed linen and maybe change the Tog value of your duvet to a lower one. Avoiding hot drinks and alcohol at bedtime may help too. Although the menopause is the most likely reason for it, now is the time to find out more about the effects of menopause, by seeing your practice nurse or GP.

I am 52 and have just started to experience irregular periods. It is my intention to 'go it alone' and try to rely on exercise and a good diet. I know that a positive attitude can be very powerful. I am an optimist but also realistic. Should I experience difficulties (e.g. hot flushes/mood swings) what would be the ONE thing I should consider taking?

I am delighted to hear about your positive mental attitude and healthy lifestyle. I wish more women approached midlife like this! Certainly increasing the amount of soya products, whole foods and calcium in your diet will be helpful, as will avoiding any dietary trigger factors such as caffeine, alcohol, spicy food and some food additives. Regular exercise has many benefits including reducing hot flushes, weight management and improving a sense of well-being.

It is hard to give you just one recommendation for hot flushes or mood swings. My main advice would be don't discount HRT completely. There are many modern low-dose HRT preparations available that can be used for a short period of time. An alternative approach is homeopathy, which can also be used to treat different physical and emotional symptoms. I would also suggest trying a general menopause supplement that includes black cohosh.

(Editor's note: see pages 71, 72 and 74 for information about safety issues and contraindications when taking black cohosh.)

In common with many of my friends, I have had problems after coming off HRT. We are all healthy women but hot flushes and night sweats have come back. What is the best way to cope?

Before coming off HRT, I ask my patients to revisit the decision that made them choose HRT initially. We look at the reasons for continuing to use it and the risks that it may present to them in their situation. Generally after two to three years of stability on HRT, I will have suggested a gradual reduction, as it is likely that symptoms can then be controlled with smaller doses. This should be done slowly to allow adjustment to occur. Coming off HRT quickly is more likely to trigger rebound symptoms. Some women manage to come off HRT with no further problems but others find that their symptoms return. Of these, some choose to cope with their symptoms, for example, avoiding caffeine and keeping alcohol to a minimum. Others try complementary or non-hormonal alternatives, bearing in mind the provisos of these therapies. Of the complementary alternatives, I would suggest black cohosh for flushes, agnus castus for mood swings and red clover as a phytoestrogen. Women need to be aware that the studies of these are less rigorous than for conventional medicine. A reputable brand should be chosen to ensure consistency and reliability of the formulation. Of the non-hormonal alternatives, the only product with evidence of benefit for flushes better than placebo is low-dose venlafaxine, a serotonin-noradrenaline reuptake inhibitor antidepressant (SNRI).

Some women make an informed decision, that the balance of risk and benefit is such that hormone therapy at the lowest effective dose to relieve symptoms is their best option. Should this be the case, the decision should be reviewed once a year or if there are any concerns.

I should like to know what I can do to help my hot flushes and night sweats apart from black cohosh, agnus castus and isoflavones?

The following strategies help with menopause symptom control. In women who need relief for mild vasomotor symptoms, first consider lifestyle changes, either alone or combined with a non-prescription remedy, such as dietary isoflavones (phytoestrogens). Herbal medicines or acupuncture have been reported as helpful for menopause symptom control but the research findings are not as good as for hormone replacement therapy (HRT). Lifestyle changes include healthy balanced diet, smoking cessation, reduced alcohol intake, exercise and stress relief. HRT remains the standard treatment for moderate to severe menopause-related hot flushes. Recommended options for women with concerns or contraindications to HRT include prescription progestogens, clonidine, the SSRI and SNRI groups of anti-depressants and gabapentin. You will need to discuss the suitability of these for yourself with your doctor. Treatment should be periodically reassessed as menopause-related vasomotor symptoms will abate over time without any intervention in most women.

My wife seems to be going through the menopause. She has hot flushes at least once a day and is often irritable. I have tried to bring up the subject but she just passes it off. How can I speak to her about her symptoms and urge her to seek help?

This needs diplomacy as well as compassion! Maybe you could say that you have noticed how uncomfortable the flushes are and would she like you to go with her to seek help? Or you could say that you have been reading about the menopause and wonder if she could tell you more about it. This might lead her into a more open discussion. Explain that you need to know more about it, to understand how she is feeling. Are there 'triggers' for her flushes or irritability? If you can identify these, you may be able to prepare for them and perhaps most of all, you can reassure her of your support. If she has a well-woman appointment soon, suggest she mentions it then.

When I came off HRT in the spring, I spent a fortune in the health shop trying to stop hot flushes to no avail. I

would like to know the best natural or herbal remedies to banish the flushes.

Alternative treatments for the relief of menopausal symptoms (e.g. phytoestrogens and black cohosh for hot flushes) have been steadily gaining popularity over the last few years. Owing to this, there are now more and more choices available for women aimed at helping a variety of menopausal symptoms. However, unlike conventional medicine there are fewer regulations governing the use of over-the-counter remedies. This means that we can't always be sure that products contain what they state. Therefore, it is very difficult to mention or suggest individual products. Small-scale studies that have been done show mixed results. Some studies find that these products do benefit symptom control, whilst others find no change in the amount of symptoms experienced. You should speak to your local pharmacist about the products available. To help with hot flushes, it may be better to choose a phytoestrogen containing all four isoflavones. These are genestein, daidzein, formononetin and biochanin. Like all medicines, some products may have side effects or contraindications, so always read the information provided. For some women, alternative medical options are available that avoid the use of HRT.

I am 51 and I have hot flushes, which are making life very difficult for me. I don't have any medical conditions and I am not taking any medication. I don't want to take HRT. What are the best alternatives?

Hot flushes can be difficult to cope with. They often go away, although they are very persistent in some women. You have told me that you have been fully investigated, but make sure you have had a thyroid function test. Certain lifestyle factors should be monitored. Avoid synthetic clothes, for example. If you do get night sweats it is best not to use a duvet, as separate layers of bedding can be removed as necessary. Coffee, tea and alcohol can also be initiating factors, so try to avoid these if you find that they stimulate a hot flush. Stress can equally be an aggravating feature. Simple yoga exercises can be helpful to relax your body. Herbal remedies are also useful, although not many studies demonstrate their benefits. I regularly recommend Menoherbs 2. Other useful complementary therapies include acupuncture and possibly reflexology.

(Editor's note: Before taking any herbal remedies or dietary supplements, check with a health professional that they are suitable for you, especially if you have a chronic medical condition or take any prescribed medicines.)

I have been getting hot flushes for six weeks now and have had disturbed sleep for that length of time which is making me irritable and tearful. I am hardly aware of them during the day but at night they usually occur regularly every two hours, and sometimes every 35 minutes when I do not get any sleep at all. I first started getting hot flushes two years ago when I was 44 and my doctor recommended incorporating soya into my diet which stopped them completely. However, they must now be more severe as the soya does not seem to be helping much. My daily intake is cereal with soya milk, 50 mg scoop of soya protein isolate powder, a soya yoghurt and a sandwich made with soya bread and sometimes a soya shake drink. My mother has advised me to reduce the amount of soya I eat as she has recently read an article in a magazine that it can be bad

for you. I do not wish to take HRT but do you think that is the only option?

Soya products can be helpful in reducing hot flushes. However, they are about 1000 times less potent than natural oestrogens. As your own oestrogen levels are dropping, the soya supplements have become less effective. The amount you eat is much more than the average British woman but not excessively high. Although phytoestrogens are generally considered safe treatments, there are few data on their safety for long-term use.

As your hot flushes are disturbing your sleep so much, I would suggest that you consider HRT for a short time, as it can reduce your hot flushes by 70-80 per cent. Obviously, you would need to check with your doctor that HRT is a suitable option for you and discuss any particular worries or fears you may have about using hormones.

If you wish to avoid HRT then other non-hormonal drug options include venlafaxine, which may reduce the flushes by 45 to 65 per cent, or gabapentin. Your GP may want you to discuss these options with a menopause specialist as they can have side effects.

I am 60 years old and have been on HRT (Premarin 0.625 milligrams) for 18 years. My doctor has advised me to come off HRT. So for the last three months I have been taking this dose every other day. As a result I am now suffering night sweats, hot flushes, palpitations, aching joints and migraines. I am also worried about the effect on my bones.

I take Candesartan 4 milligrams (one tablet a day for

high blood pressure) and levothyroxine 100 micrograms (one tablet a day for an underactive thyroid). I also take simvastatin 40 milligrams (one at night for cholesterol), Maxalt 10 milligrams (one or two tablets when necessary for migraine), the beta-blocker bisoprolol 5 milligrams (one tablet a day) and the diuretic bendroflumethiazide 2.5 milligrams (one tablet a day). To help keep my joints supple, I take glucosamine sulphate tablets and also cod liver oil capsules. Can you suggest anything that will help to lessen my symptoms and that will not interact with my medications?

When a decision is made to come off HRT, or oestrogen replacement therapy in your case, you should gradually come off the hormones, as otherwise you get rebound hot flushes and night sweats, which can prove to be quite troublesome. Rather then using the 0.625 milligram Premarin dose on alternate days, try taking the 'half dose' tablet (Premarin 0.3 milligrams) daily for around three months and then stop. If your Premarin 0.625 milligram tablets are scored, then you could cut the tablets in half and then take half a tablet daily. If they are sugar-coated then it will not be easy to cut the tablets in half. In this case, your pharmacist can try to get you Premarin 0.3 milligrams. Of course you will have to ask your GP for a prescription first. You need to be aware that it could take between three to four months after stopping your Premarin before you settle and are finally symptom free. This can be the case whether you stop the 0.625 milligram dose now or after using the 0.3 milligram dose for three months. So another option would be to stop your Premarin 0.625 milligram tablets now and give yourself three months' settling time.

With regards to good symptom control, we know, for example,

that patients with uncontrolled blood pressure or with thyroid problems can also get hot flushes and night sweats. So you need to make sure you have got good control by taking your blood pressure and thyroxine tablets regularly and having checks as your GP recommends. You can also help yourself by doing breathing and stretching exercises, and generally looking after yourself by having a healthy balanced diet as well.

There are herbal treatments that can help with hot flushes and night sweats. You need to be careful with black cohosh and sage, as these could affect your blood pressure medications. You could try taking red clover tablets (you can buy these from a health food store or a pharmacy) or eating more soya-based foods, for example soya milk or yoghurts. These are dietary sources of plant-type oestrogen, which can help with symptom control.

With regards to bone health, good calcium and vitamin D intake is necessary. This can come from your diet or you can take supplements. For a comprehensive risk assessment for osteoporosis and fracture prevention, you need to speak with your doctor, who will help you decide how to manage now that you are coming off oestrogen replacement therapy.

I am going through the menopause. I work five days a week in an office and find that by mid-afternoon my energy levels drop. Can you suggest ways to increase my energy levels?

This is a common difficulty, whether you are going through the menopause or not. You could look at your eating habits, ensuring that you are eating regularly and avoiding sugary snacks, which often have only a short-lived effect. Keep your weight under control and try to get out into the fresh air when you have a break. If allowed, small frequent breaks can be useful. In the long term, taking regular exercise and ensuring a healthy balanced diet will help to improve your vitality. Many women going through the menopause suffer from hot flushes and night sweats. If these symptoms are affecting your sleep, then this can be a reason for low energy levels noted during the course of the day.

I am going through quite severe menopausal problems. I had anorexia nervosa from my late teens to my early thirties. My periods re-started in my mid-thirties after having hormone treatment. I have had eczema since having hormone treatment but it is now worse. I am 56. For the last two years my monthly cycle has been irregular. I now have increasingly dry skin on my body and scalp and have dry eyes. My hair is falling out. I suffer from gum bleeds with blood in my mouth, particularly at night. I have severe wind and discomfort in my bowels and diarrhoea. I have weakness in my legs and severe depression at times.

I am not on any medication. I tried 0.625 micrograms Prempak 18 months ago but it didn't suit me. I have tried homeopathy. I saw a nutritionist and have tried supplements including soya capsules and have used soya milk etc (but not red clover).

Do you suggest that I try another HRT product and if so, which one? What else do you suggest?

Because of your anorexia nervosa for about 20 years you are unfortunately at high risk of osteoporosis. I think you need to go back to your GP and ask for a referral to a specialist menopause clinic; there are regional referral centres around the country, and someone with as complex a story as yours really deserves super-specialist consideration (i.e. not just a gynaecologist, but a gynaecologist with a specialist interest in the menopause and osteoporosis). For example, you are one of the few people in your 50s who should have a DEXA scan for bone density. Only when you have that information can you make an informed decision about possible treatments for your wellbeing and bones.

There are plenty of other HRT preparations that might suit you better, and with dry skin and hair loss I always check with a blood test to exclude an underactive thyroid too. Red clover is excellent, but just may not be enough for you. Have courage and go back to your GP for another consultation.

Which herbs and supplements would best help vaginal symptoms?

There is very little information available from clinical trials and therefore very little evidence to support the use of herbs and supplements to help specifically with vaginal symptoms at the time of the menopause. However, there are a few small studies that have looked at alternative treatments.

A USA study[21] on 100 women found that women using HRT and dietary supplements such as soy, ginkgo biloba and black cohosh reported greater improvement in vaginal dryness, libido (sex drive) and mood compared with women using HRT alone. An Australian study[22] looked at the effect of soy-protein dietary supplements in healthy postmenopausal women. Ninety-four older postmenopausal women with a high frequency of mild menopausal symptoms took soy supplements for three months and were compared with a group of 100 women who did not take any soy supplements. There was no difference in symptom control, such as hot flushes and night sweats, between the two groups. However, interestingly, the first group found that they had a significant improvement in vaginal dryness, whereas this was not the case in the women in the second group who were taking dummy treatment.

For vaginal dryness, you can use lubricants, such as KY Jelly or Astroglide. Isoflavone vaginal creams are also available, but it is not clear whether the associated improvement is due to their lubricant-type ingredients or the isoflavone component. Women with vaginal symptoms can also discuss with their doctor whether a prescription for vaginal oestrogen preparations (available as creams, pessaries, vaginal tablets or rings) will be helpful.

Since being on HRT there has been a dramatic drop in my libido. I have tried many herbal supplements that claim to help, but with no success. Is there anything that you can recommend to help me?

Firstly, it is important to check whether vaginal dryness is affecting your libido. If so, this can be easily remedied with vaginal oestrogen preparations, (creams, pessaries, vaginal tablets and rings). Secondly, the need for counselling should be considered, as lifestyle stresses and relationship problems can affect libido. What type of HRT is being taken should also be considered, as this can be adjusted to improve low libido. Assess all the medicines you are on, to check if one has a side effect that impacts on libido. If you still find that libido is a problem, then your doctor may assess you for a testosterone implant. This provides a small level of male hormone, and is licensed to relieve low libido after the menopause. For an assessment, you will need to see your doctor for referral to a specialist clinic at your local hospital.

I seem to be coping with the menopause quite well, using soya isoflavones to help with the hot flushes. I have a healthy lifestyle, eating- and exercise-wise. I am not on any medication. I'm 56 years old and I last had a period 14 months ago. Basically sex is very painful. Even having a recent smear test (and the nurse used a smaller instrument) was difficult and painful. I consulted my GP a few months ago about this and she tried me on Ovestin cream, which I applied regularly as prescribed. This does not appear to have made a huge difference. All of this obviously doesn't help my libido!! Please can you give me advice on how to cope with my problem. Are there any other prescription drugs that might help?

There are prescription medicines that can be used to help with menopausal libido problems. For this, you would need a full menopause review, with clinical assessment to ensure there is no other cause. Generally, after trying local vaginal oestrogen creams, pessaries or tablets, the next stage would be to assess whether systemic HRT (taken by mouth or used as a patch system for example) plus or minus testosterone replacement therapy may be required. At the same time, any simultaneous lifestyle or psychosexual issues that may be having an effect on your libido would be addressed by a referral for counselling support. If you were to decide not to take systemic HRT, then the only immediate option is to try other local formulations of oestrogen to see if these are more helpful.

How much exercise do you recommend for women at the menopause?

All of us should be exercising, whether we are menopausal or not. Exercise is an important part of keeping healthy, along with maintaining a balanced diet. Regular exercise is better than occasional strenuous bouts and it does not need to hurt to be beneficial. Building exercise into your daily pattern of life is essential. Some people like to take their exercise in classes for support and enjoyment. Others will enjoy country walks or sports. Anyone who has not exercised for a while should see their GP prior to starting an exercise programme. When built into your daily life exercise can be difficult to measure but about 20 minutes brisk exercise three times a week is said to be beneficial. Walking is the easiest thing to do: aim for 30 minutes, five days per week.

I am 48 and I am finding it difficult to give up smoking. What effect will smoking have on my menopause? I have heard that smoking can affect my bones. Is this true?

Firstly, well done for trying to give up smoking and don't stop trying. It's worth asking your GP for help, because your local smoking cessation team will be able to give you individualised support. Your local pharmacist may also be able to help. Smoking and being childless are related to an early menopause and a shorter perimenopause (the time from the beginning of irregular periods until one year after the last period) because the eggs in the ovaries of smokers run out sooner. Smokers also have lower levels of the female hormone oestradiol, which can result in a higher chance of developing osteoporosis (brittle bones) in later life. It is important to look after your bones by eating a healthy diet with plenty of calcium-rich food, maintaining an optimal weight and taking regular weight-bearing exercise like running, tennis or aerobics.

Which alternative remedies work best for mood swings and anxiety?

Remember HALT: do not get Hungry, Angry, Lonely or Tired. Self-help is essential. Remember to do plenty of exercise, ideally 20-30 minutes a day but the more the better. Do not forget to get out in the daylight for at least an hour in each day and eat well. Taking warm to hot baths with aromatherapy oils for 20 minutes can also help as can learning relaxation techniques such as meditation or yoga. Any alternative medicine must be discussed with your health professionals and if you want to go down the alternative route it may be a good idea to see an appropriately trained and qualified CAM practitioner. Two registers to look at include the International Register of Consultant Herbalists and Homeopaths, and the National Institute of Medical Herbalists. St John's Wort has been beneficial but one needs to be careful about interaction with other drugs that you may be on. If self-help has not worked it is important to go to discuss it with your medical doctor because drug therapy may be required.

Chapter 8

Women's Health and General Health Issues

The Menopause Exchange was set up to provide information about the menopause and related topics. But we have found that many of our members want to know more about other health topics as diverse as breast cancer, fibroids, carpal tunnel syndrome, myalgic encephalomyelitis (ME) and snoring.

Some of these medical conditions or symptoms are more common in women over 50, while others can affect women (and men) at any time of their life. There are also certain conditions (e.g. diabetes) that affect how a woman's menopausal symptoms are treated. If you experience any new symptoms, don't just assume that they are due to the menopause. You should always seek medical advice, just to be sure.

***

Breast cancer

What is the best option for women with menopausal symptoms who have had breast cancer?

There is no easy answer to this. Most women will not be offered HRT if they have had breast cancer, and non-hormonal therapies are not always effective. Some women use complementary therapies with good effect, others rely on lifestyle management (e.g. identify things which trigger hot flushes and reduce them accordingly). Vaginal dryness can often be treated with local oestrogen creams even if you have had breast cancer, because when the creams are used at an appropriate dose, they are not absorbed into the blood stream. For hot flushes, progestogen may be prescribed to some women or clonidine (a non-hormonal treatment) may be suitable. Other medical treatments such as venlafaxine and gabapentin may be suggested, but usually referral to a specialist unit is necessary.

I had to stop taking HRT when the investigations began that led to my breast cancer being diagnosed. I do miss it, as my memory, concentration and confidence have suffered. I have gone to a homeopath and wonder what natural preparations you would suggest to replace HRT?

You are making the same assumption that many women make – that 'natural' treatments must be safe to use after breast cancer. Some of the 'natural' treatments work much like oestrogen, so may not be recommended for women who have had breast cancer. That said, you could try black cohosh or gingko biloba, both of which claim to relieve menopausal complaints and are not thought to affect the breast. Some Bach flower remedies claim to aid concentration and memory and are unlikely to be harmful. If you have had breast cancer (or any other cancer), check with your breast cancer nurse or doctor before starting any new treatments, natural or conventional, just to be sure.

I am 53 years old and have been through my menopause. I have had breast cancer and I am now taking tamoxifen tablets. Since taking them, I have been experiencing hot flushes and night sweats. What can I do to ease these?

Tamoxifen is commonly associated with severe menopausal symptoms, which can often be worse than the symptoms experienced with a natural menopause. HRT is very effective at reducing hot flushes but its use is controversial after breast cancer. Non-hormonal alternatives include some antidepressants, which can be very helpful and have no adverse effect on breast cancer recurrence rates. Venlafaxine and fluoxetine are two examples which can reduce hot flushes by 50 to 60 per cent. I recommend talking to your breast surgeon before making this very personal decision about recurrence risk versus quality of life.

I had breast cancer three years ago and I am taking tamoxifen which is giving me hot flushes. What options do I have for dealing with these?

Lifestyle issues are always important to address in this situation. Self-help is obviously the first way to approach this. Avoid known triggers including hot spicy foods, chocolate and alcohol. Stress can also induce a hot flush so try to minimise this. Breathing exercises, including alternate nostril breathing, can help you to relax. It is important to ditch polyester, nylon or other man-made fibres in your wardrobe as these trap the heat and make flushes much worse. Don't forget to have an electric fan because that can often help. Never get dehydrated and drink plenty of still cool water. Using other remedies including phytoestrogens can be considered. It is essential that you discuss this with your oncologist because we want to make sure that everybody works in an integrated rather than an isolated way. Therapies including acupuncture and hypnotherapy, where you can learn self-hypnosis, can help hot flushes.

Hysterectomy

I am having a hysterectomy soon. What will happen during the recovery period? How will the hysterectomy affect me? Can I expect to put on weight afterwards? How can I best cope?

It partly depends on why you are having the hysterectomy (e.g. cancer, prolapse, pelvic floor repair, fibroids or heavy periods), how old you are (pre or post menopause), and, if you are young, whether you are also having your ovaries removed. In other words, it is a complex situation that you must talk through with your own gynaecologist and GP, to relate the information to your specific set of circumstances. A laparoscopic hysterectomy has a shorter recovery time (two to four weeks) than an abdominal hysterectomy (six to 12 weeks), providing there are no complications like infections or blood clots. You should plan to be off work for four to 12 weeks, depending on how physically demanding your job is. Fill your freezer now! You can usually drive after four to six weeks (later if an abdominal wound as this takes time to heal). Some women do put on weight, but not everyone. Plan a healthy diet high in fruit and vegetables and get back to exercising as soon as is reasonably possible. (Check with your doctor first.) The Hysterectomy Association offers information and advice.

Fibroids

I am 47 and I have fibroids. Will they be affected by the menopause?

Yes. Fibroids are benign lumpy bits of muscle that grow inside the uterus, on its outside or in its walls. They can affect the way your uterus contracts, making periods heavier. Occasionally, fibroids can get so big that they can actually cause problems with bladder emptying. Virtually all older women have them. Fibroids are hormone sensitive, so the great news is that at the menopause they shrivel up. If you have large fibroids and take HRT, however, they can be stimulated to grow even larger, and this requires regular assessment by the prescribing doctor.

I am 52 years old and I was first diagnosed with fibroids following surgery to remove a benign growth from my cervix in the early 90s. For most of the time, they have been a 'bearable discomfort' but, in the past six months or so, they have become very painful. My GP ordered an ultrasound scan, which showed my uterus to be 'lumpy', but a full blood screen showed absolutely no problems whatsoever. Nevertheless she referred me to a gynaecologist who decided upon examining me to 'leave well alone' as I should, in theory, be close to the menopause, although there is no sign of that so far. She told me that fibroids shrink away almost to nothing when the menopause occurs. But in the meantime – what do I do? The only symptom I have is the pain. What advice can you give me?

Your doctors have done the right tests to investigate your fibroid uterus (womb), but don't seem to appreciate the pain you are experiencing. Your uterus is not particularly enlarged ('lumpy' means lots of small fibroids were seen on the ultrasound scan) and your periods are not heavy enough to make you anaemic. Therefore there is no pressing need to offer you a hysterectomy, the permanent solution to a fibroid uterus. A hysterectomy is a major operation and should only be undertaken for carefully considered reasons. The average age for the menopause, the final natural period, for women in the UK, is about 51 years of age, and over 80 per cent of women have had their menopause by age 54. So, your doctors are correct, you should be nearly there!

Besides a hysterectomy or a myomectomy (the operation that just removes the fibroids but leaves the uterus intact) there are other possible medical treatments. These would aim to 'switch off' your periods to prevent the fibroids from growing any more and reduce your pain. The most effective and well-established treatment (an injection of goserelin) makes women temporarily menopausal. It may seem a bit drastic when you are so close to the natural menopause, and it can cause significant bone loss. Another approach would be to suppress ovulation in your natural menstrual cycle with a hormone, such as desogestrel. Or you could rely on regular doses of an anti-inflammatory painkiller, which can be very effective for period pain.

I suggest that you return to your GP or the consultant to explain the pain that you are experiencing and discuss possible treatments.

Endometriosis

My daughter has endometriosis. Please can you tell me about it? How can it be treated?

All women have endometriosis to some extent or other. If you look inside a woman's abdominal cavity for any reason, you can see it, but what doctors don't understand is why some women get symptoms of severe pain and/or infertility and others don't.

Endometriosis is the normal lining (endometrium) of the uterus, or womb, growing in other places. At a period, the lining is shed and mainly drops out (vaginal bleeding), but as you lie down to sleep, some trickles back down your Fallopian tubes and spills into your abdominal cavity. The endometrial cells may then take root and grow into little cysts that still think they are in the uterus; these still follow the menstrual cycle each month, growing and then bleeding. This is why some women get pain in their abdomen (often radiating down the legs) just before a period, as these endometrial cysts are at their largest. As the period ends, the cysts deflate and the pain gets better. Patches of endometrium can be stuck on your gut, giving bowel symptoms, or bladder, causing bladder irritation. They can block the Fallopian tubes or ovary, causing infertility.

There are many treatment options that a specialist gynaecologist can offer, mostly giving hormones to block the normal cycle, so the cysts are not stimulated. Pregnancy is a brilliant treatment, but may not be a practical solution. The Mirena intrauterine coil is another very useful option, or taking the contraceptive pill continuously without a break. At the menopause, endometriosis regresses. Endometriosis UK is a charity providing information and support.

Miscellaneous problems

I have a double chamber uterus. What effect, if any, would that have on my menopause (regarding bleeding)? Please can you give me some advice?

Double chamber wombs are rare, and women are born with them. Usually when a fetus's reproductive organs are forming, two tubes come together to form the uterus or womb. (Their top separate ends form the Fallopian tubes.) As they stick together, the middle wall dissolves, forming a larger chamber. Sometimes, (in your case, for example), this wall is left, so you get a 'bicornuate uterus', which looks like a V. Some women can have two vaginas, but this is very rare. This mainly causes problems with pregnancy, but no problems whatever at the menopause. Possibly you may have always bled more than other women, as your uterus has twice the surface area (get your GP to check you for iron deficiency). The good news is that at the menopause the periods stop.

It is two years since my last period – is a blood test helpful to assess hormones levels?

The very last bleed that you have represents your menopause, but you will not know this until you have waited a year. If you are over 45 and your last natural period was two years ago, you are by definition postmenopausal. Blood tests will add little to this, particularly if you are experiencing hot flushes and night sweats and other symptoms associated with low oestrogen levels. You can be advised about your personal risk factors and the benefits and risks of any intervention without any further investigations being necessary. If you are less than 45 and particularly in the absence of symptoms, blood tests will help to identify the cause of your lack of periods. Ovarian failure leading to menopause can then be considered from among the list of other potential causes.

My local pharmacy offers blood pressure and cholesterol testing. How accurate is this? I would like to have mine checked, but am I better off seeing my GP or practice nurse rather than a pharmacist?

Like other diagnostic services, blood pressure monitoring and cholesterol testing are now offered by certain pharmacies. The equipment used by the pharmacists is very advanced and is actually identical to those used by GP surgeries. The blood pressure monitors these days provide accurate digital readings. However, it is crucial to keep in mind that any cholesterol tests done through a pharmacy are random tests, with no control over fat on unclean hands or the content and time of your previous meals. The cholesterol level detected is only a guide, and you should be referred to your GP if it is high. The pharmacist may discuss lifestyle and diet changes with you if necessary. The advantage of seeing your pharmacist for diagnostic tests such as these is that you don't have to make an appointment with your GP or practice nurse.

I am 54 and have recently started taking low-dose HRT (Kliovance) to relieve my sleeping problems. I have experienced menopausal symptoms for about seven years and have not had any periods for about 13 months. I

don't want to stay on HRT for any longer than I have to. I just want to know if it does help with sleeping problems. Also, if I stay on it for about two years, are my symptoms likely to have stopped by then anyway? I am also taking valerian to help with sleep and want to know if it is OK to continue taking this.

Sleep disturbance is a genuine problem that occurs at or after the menopause and is due to oestrogen deficiency. It causes waking with an active mind in the small hours and is different from an anxiety attack or night sweats. In some women, sleep disturbance may continue after the sweats have spontaneously settled. The length of time that these problems last varies and it is impossible to predict.

For many, oestrogen replacement is helpful as it deals with the cause of the disturbance. It is however important to exclude anxiety, depression, pain or other causes of sleeplessness, as they will need a different approach.

Valerian is a very mild sedative that doesn't appear addictive. However, you have to make sure that valerian doesn't slow your essential reaction times, for example when driving; otherwise, the herb can be regarded as safe.

I am 53 and I started my menopause at the age of 45. I spent five years on HRT, which were pretty uneventful – no hot flushes or night sweats. I came off HRT at 50 because I didn't want to prolong taking the tablets, but I ended up with all the symptoms again, which are now subsiding if I watch what I eat and drink. My main problem now is snoring which started about two years ago. I

am not sure if this is a result of my age, the menopause, my weight (although I am not excessively overweight) or a hereditary problem. Could it be due to any of these? Is there anything I can do to stop snoring without resorting to an operation?

Snoring occurs when a lax soft palate acts as a sounding board as you breathe in and out. If your partner says you have long pauses between snores, get referred by your GP to a 'sleep clinic'. There is a serious condition called 'sleep apnoea' where you actually stop breathing in the night for short periods of time, so your oxygen levels plummet and you wake up feeling tired and groggy. Usually sleep apnoeics are grossly overweight, and may drink too much. Alcohol relaxes the soft palate and makes you snore, while smokers snore twice as often as non-smokers.

In the post-menopause your collagen gets looser everywhere, so it's logical to think we snore more, but I don't think anyone has looked at it. A blocked nose from an allergy or polyps also makes you a snoring mouth breather, as does sleeping on your back, rather than on your side. If your nose is blocked, consult your GP for an ear, nose and throat (ENT) referral.

There are plastic gum shields that slightly move your jaw to tighten your soft palate as you sleep. For further information contact the British Snoring & Sleep Apnoea Association.

I suffer from painful periods. What can I buy from a pharmacy that will help this?

Period pains are caused by contractions in the muscles of the uterus, which are triggered by hormones produced by the lining of the uterus. Painkillers from a pharmacy will help with the discomfort. Most of these contain paracetamol, ibuprofen or aspirin, alone or in combination with codeine or dihydrocodeine. Some products, such as Feminax Period Pain Capsules, are a combination treatment especially formulated for period pain, although the formula is similar to other pain relief medications. It is crucial that you seek advice from the pharmacist for the most appropriate combination for you. If you are sensitive to aspirin or ibuprofen, for example, you may only be able to take paracetamol. If these painkillers don't help, ask your pharmacist about Feminax Ultra, which is now available over the counter from pharmacies – this contains the stronger painkiller naproxen, which reduces the contractions of the uterus. Naproxen was previously available on prescription only. Using a hot water bottle with any medication will ease the pain. If the pharmacy-strength products don't help, you should consult your GP. Prescribed medication may be needed for severe period pain.

Can the menopause be linked to carpal tunnel syndrome? Do you have any suggestions for getting rid of it besides surgery?

Patients can present with carpal tunnel syndrome (pain, tingling and weakness in the middle fingers, from compression of the median nerve as it goes though the wrist) at the menopause. If women choose to take HRT, carpal tunnel syndrome improves, only to return when HRT is stopped. You can buy elastic wrist splints from pharmacies and sleep in them, to take the pressure off the wrist. Also a steroid injection into the tunnel usually reduces inflammation, creating more room for the nerve, often improving symptoms for three to six months. Your

GP may inject your wrist or refer you to someone who can do it. Surgery does cure the problem forever and can be done under local anaesthetic, but you won't be able to drive or use your hand properly for about a month.

Do ME symptoms increase at the menopause?

ME (myalgic encephalomyelitis/encephalopathy) is a chronic, fluctuating illness also known as chronic fatigue syndrome (CFS) or post viral fatigue syndrome (PVFS). The illness affects many parts of the body, such as the nervous and immune systems. The most common symptoms are severe fatigue or exhaustion, problems with memory and concentration and muscle pain. The cause or causes of ME are not fully understood. It often develops after a virus, like flu or glandular fever, but it can also happen gradually for no obvious reason. The menopause is not a cause of ME, but for some women, menopausal symptoms may be similar to those described in ME, such as tiredness, poor memory and concentration and joint pains. This means it may be difficult to know what is causing which symptoms, if you already have symptoms of ME. You will need to discuss this with your doctor, along with strategies for relieving the effects of menopause.

Does the menopause have any effect on asthma?

In my clinical practice, I have not noticed that the menopause increases or worsens asthma symptoms. I have been unable to find any scientific evidence that the menopause has any significant effect on (pre-existing) asthma. However, oestrogen and progestogen HRT may increase the chance of developing asthma and asthma-like symptoms, such as wheezing, in a small number of women.

Do allergies increase at the menopause?

An allergy is your immune system's abnormal reaction if you come into contact with a specific substance (called an allergen). The chemicals released cause the sneezing, rash, irritation and other allergy symptoms. Generally speaking, the menopause itself does not cause allergies. However, individual women do report a change in some symptoms, such as hay fever or asthma, during the hormonal upset of the menopause, just as they do during other hormonal changes, such as puberty or pregnancy. It is unclear why this might be the case and you should seek medical advice if necessary.

I am 50 and I am going through the menopause. When I was young I suffered from acne. For the last few months I have been getting spots on my face. Does acne worsen at the menopause? What products can I buy from a pharmacy to help this condition?

Acne is one of the symptoms of the menopause. Some women who haven't had a spot since their teens find themselves coming out with acne. Like the teenage years, the menopause involves hormone changes, which cause the skin to produce more oil, clogging up the pores of the skin. Bacteria start to build up and inflammation sets in, with white pus accumulating.

A healthy well-balanced diet is crucial in combating acne, to-gether with drinking plenty of water. A routine of cleansing and exfoliating your skin will remove the dead layer of cells, reducing the blockage of pores. Pharmacies sell acne products for mild to moderate acne. Apply the products to the entire area, not just to the spots. All products take weeks to work – so be patient. For severe acne, seek the advice of your GP for stronger prescription medication.

Resist picking or squeezing spots. Take care with hygiene; simple washing with an anti-bacterial soap and warm water will help to manage the condition. If the condition has not improved after eight weeks of over-the-counter products, or if the condition worsens, then speak to your doctor.

Appendix

HRT and breast cancer risk

The association between HRT (oestrogen and progestogen) and breast cancer is probably the one issue that causes the greatest concern to women and health professionals. It is important to remember that the risk for breast cancer increases as women age. A large meta-analysis published in 1997 showed that for every 1000 women not taking HRT, the background population risk at age 50 was around 45; that is 45 women per 1000 will get breast cancer. By age 60, this figure goes up to 51 women, and by age 70, up to 57 per 1000 women. Therefore it is very important that women between the ages of 50 and 70 attend for mammograms every three years, as offered by the UK NHS Breast Screening Programme.

Women often say that having their breasts pressed between screening plates is painful, and that this puts them off having mammograms. However, it may be the case that a mammogram will identify a breast lump early on and, with treatment, the woman has the chance of a near-normal life span. Thinking of mammograms in this context may make women feel that it is worth bearing the pain for the two to three minutes whilst their breasts are being x-rayed. In-between having mammograms, women should also be doing breast self-examinations. In this way, women can help themselves by keeping an eye out for any breast changes that may occur and which should be reported as early as possible to their doctors.

HRT and breast cancer risk

Trying to work out the absolute (true) risk of breast cancer with HRT use is very difficult. Experts still don't know whether oestrogen and progestogen actually cause breast cancer or whether they act as promoters (accelerating an already-existing tumour so that the cancer is seen earlier than would have been otherwise).

Findings from studies suggest that HRT taken for more than five years results in an additional risk to the age-related risk discussed above, but that this overall risk is lower if only oestrogen is used. However, for women who have not had a hysterectomy (surgical removal of the uterus), oestrogen should not be taken on its own. Progestogen plays an important role in women with an intact uterus by protecting the uterine lining and preventing endometrial cancer.

The Million Women Study

A UK trial that studied over a million women suggested that HRT may increase the risk for breast cancer after as little as a year after starting HRT. These findings have been challenged, as the women were asked to fill in a 10-page general health questionnaire when coming in for a mammogram; when a quarter of the forms were checked against GP records, the information provided was not factually correct. However, because large numbers of women were involved, and most of the data were correct, it has been useful to note that this study also indicated the highest risk with combined HRT, with a lower risk for women using oestrogen-only products. Livial ('no-bleed' HRT) came somewhere in the middle between 'combined HRT' and 'oestrogen only' for additional breast cancer risk. It has also been suggested that the breast cancer cases seen in women after as little as one year could be due to previous usage of HRT before joining the study.

Women's Health Initiative Study
The US-based WHI study assessed 16,608 women between the ages of 50 to 79. This randomised controlled trial provides us with the best information available to date, although there still remain many unanswered questions. The WHI investigators reported a significant 26% increase in the relative increase for invasive breast cancer in women taking combined HRT over five years. In terms of numbers of women affected, this is an actual increased risk for 8 more per 1000 women. They also noted that the longer HRT was taken, the higher the breast cancer risk. As the average age of women in this study was 63, another ongoing medical debate is around the question of whether the five-year breast cancer risk applies to women who take HRT more than 10 years after going through the menopause as opposed to starting at the menopausal age of around 50.

Analysis of the WHI group of women who had had hysterectomies and took oestrogen only HRT for over seven years showed some surprising results. In this group, it was noted that there was a reduction in the numbers of breast cancers and even in heart risk. The results were not significant, that is the statistical tests applied could not show whether this was by chance or whether it was a true finding. There is a need for more research in this area.

Current consensus
Women on HRT should be assessed every year in view of new

knowledge and changing risk factors. Based on the information available, and bearing in mind that most women will use HRT for menopause symptom control and after an individualised risk-benefit evaluation, it is felt that HRT benefits generally outweigh risks for women between 50 to 59. However, after the age of 60, the risks may start to outweigh the benefits.

In healthy women with menopausal symptoms who need HRT when they are going through or have just gone through their menopause in their early 50s, the benefits (including possible protection of the heart) may outweigh the risks. These women could consider using HRT for up to five years, or even up to the age of 60. After this, they should be advised slowly to come off HRT, as breast cancer, stroke and thrombosis risks increase with age and, for breast cancer, the length of time HRT is used. Women may accept the higher risks after the age of 60 and may wish to continue HRT after discussing the benefits and risks with their doctor. Some women with breast cancer may also opt for HRT if tumour tissue studies show that their type of cancer was not oestrogen-receptor positive, making the decision after a discussion with their doctors and consultant oncologists.

*(Editor's Note: This article by **Dr Nuttan Tanna** first appeared in* **The Menopause Exchange Newsletter** *in 2008 and has been reviewed for any relevant updates for this book. Dr Nuttan Tanna is a consultant pharmacist specialising in the menopause and osteoporosis, based at The Northwick Park Menopause Clinical and Research Unit at NW London Hospitals in Harrow, Middlesex.)*

Glossary

Amenorrhoea
The absence or stopping of the menstrual periods

Anaemia
Reduction in the quantity of the oxygen-carrying pigment (haemoglobin) in the blood

Anticoagulant
A drug that prevents the clotting of blood

Auto-immune reaction
An immune reaction in which the body attacks healthy tissue, mistaking it for a foreign antigen

Beta-blocker
A drug that works to control abnormal heart rhythms, to treat angina and to reduce high blood pressure

Bone density
Measurement of the bone's mass in relation to its volume

Carpal tunnel syndrome
A combination of pins and needles, numbness and pain in the hand, usually affecting the thumb, index and middle fingers, caused by pressure on the median nerve as it passes through the wrist

Caucasian
Light or white-skinned race

Cervical spondylosis
A spinal condition resulting from degeneration and flattening of the intervertebral discs in the cervical (neck) region

Cholesterol
A fat-like material present in blood and most tissues

Coeliac disease
A condition in which the small intestine fails to digest and absorb food

Collagen
A type of protein that connects and supports other bodily tissues

Conjugated equine oestrogen
An oestrogen used in HRT which is obtained from mares' urine

Corticosteroids
Hormones produced naturally by the adrenal glands

Cyopreservation
Freezing of ovarian tissue

Diabetic
Having a medical condition in which the amount of glucose (sugar) in the blood is too high because the body can't use it properly

Dual energy x-ray absorptiometry (DEXA)
Method of measuring bone density

Electrocardiogram (ECG)
The tracing of the electrical activity of the heart recorded by electrocardiography

Endometriosis
A condition in which fragments of the lining of the uterus grow outside the uterus (womb)

Endometrium
Uterus (womb) lining

Endometrial Hyperplasia
A thickening of the lining of the uterus, caused by overgrowth of the cells that line the uterus

Fallopian tubes
Tubes which lead from the ovaries into the uterus

Fibroid
Benign tumour of fibrous tissue and muscular tissue, one or more of which may develop within or attached to the outside of the uterus

Follicle Stimulating Hormone (FSH)
One of the female hormones produced by the pituitary gland

Gingivitis
Inflammation of the gums caused by plaque on the surfaces of the teeth

Glucocorticoid
A type of corticosteroid

Grave's disease
A thyroid disorder

Haemoglobin
A substance contained within
the red blood cells

Hormone assay
A test or trial to determine
the strength of hormones

Hyperthyroidism
An overactive thyroid gland

Hyperparathyroidism
An overactive parathyroid
gland

Hyperventilation
Breathing at an abnormally
rapid rate at rest

Hysterectomy
Operation to remove the
uterus

**Irritable bowel
syndrome (IBS)**
A condition in which
recurrent abdominal pain
with constipation and/or
diarrhoea continues for years
without any general dete-
rioration in physical health

Implants
Small pellets inserted under
the skin

**Inflammatory
Arthritides**
Diseases of the joints

**Laparoscopic
Hysterectomy**
An operation to remove the
uterus through four small
cuts on the abdomen below
the navel

Libido
Sexual drive

Mammogram
A breast X-ray

ME
Myalgic Encephalopathy,
also known as Myalgic
Encephalomyelitis

Menopause
The occurrence of the
last natural menstrual
period

Neurotransmitter
A chemical substance
released from nerve endings
to transmit impulses across to
other nerves

Oestrogen
A female sex hormone
produced by the ovaries

Osteoarthritis
A degenerative disease of the
joints resulting from wear of
the articular cartilage

Osteopenia
A degree of bone loss less
severe than osteoporosis

Osteoporosis
Loss of bone tissue, resulting in bones that are brittle and liable to fracture

Ovaries
A pair of female sex glands which produce sex hormones and release eggs

Palpitations
An awareness of the heartbeat

Pelvic floor
Spans the area under the pelvis

Perimenopause
The time from the beginning of irregular periods until 12 months after the last period

Pessary
A device which fits into the vagina

Phytoestrogens
Natural plant oestrogens

Placebo
A dummy treatment

Platelet
A disc-shaped cell structure that is present in the blood

Polymyalgia rheumatica
A rheumatic disease causing aching and progressive stiffness of the muscles of the shoulders and hips after inactivity

Polyp
A growth, usually benign, protruding from a mucous membrane

Post-menopause
The stage when menstruation has not occurred for a least 12 months

Premenstrual syndrome (PMS)
A group of symptoms experienced in varying degrees by women of reproductive age in the week before menstruation

Progesterone
A female sex hormone produced by the ovaries during the second half of the menstrual cycle

Progestogen
The synthetic form of progesterone

Prolapse
Downward displacement of an organ or tissue from its normal position

Rheumatoid arthritis
An autoimmune disease that causes chronic inflammation of the joints

Rosacea
A chronic inflammatory disease of the face in which the skin becomes abnormally flushed

Sebaceous gland
Any of the simple or branched glands in the skin that secrete an oily substance

SNRIs
A class of antidepressants known as serotonin norepinephrine re-uptake inhibitors

SSRIs
A class of antidepressants known as selective serotonin re-uptake inhibitors

Sub-total thyroidectomy
Surgical removal of 90 per cent of the thyroid gland

Surgical menopause
A menopause caused by removal of the uterus

Supraventricular Tachycardia (SVT)
A rapid regular heart beat

Systemic
Relating to or affecting the body as a whole

Tachyphylaxis
Where levels of oestrogen in the blood system are too high, as a result of too many oestrogen implants over time

Testosterone
A steroid hormone formed by the ovary and adrenal glands

Thyroid gland
A large endocrine gland situated in the base of the neck that manufactures hormones and secretes them directly into the bloodstream

Thyroid stimulating antibodies
Antibodies that stimulate the thyroid gland

Thyroidectomy
Surgical removal of the thyroid gland

Tog-value
The international standard measurement of all blankets' thermal effectiveness

Urethra
The opening of the bladder

Uterus
A female organ which holds the developing unborn child. Also called the womb

Vagina
The lower part of the female reproductive tract

Vaginal atrophy
Inflammation of the vagina and the outer urinary tract

Vasomotor symptoms
Symptoms caused by the irregular function of the part of the brain that controls body heat (such as hot flushes and night sweats)

Vertigo
A disabling sensation in which the affected individual feels that either he himself or his surroundings are in a state of constant movement

Withdrawal bleed
The breaking down of the lining of the uterus and shedding after stopping a course of progestogen

Womb
Also called the uterus

References

1. Gupta P, Sturdee DW, Hunter MS. Mid-age health in women from the Indian subcontinent (MAHWIS): general health and the experience of menopause in women. *Climacteric* 2006; 9(1):13-22.

2. Sethi K, Pitkin J. British-Asian women's views on and attitudes towards menopause and hormone replacement therapy. 2000; 3(4):248-253.

3. Hunter M. Cognitive behavioural interventions for premenstrual and menopause symptoms. *Journal of Reproduction & Infant Psychology* 2003; 21:183-193.

4. Rotem M, Kushnir T, Levine R, Ehrenfeld M. A Psycho-Educational Program for Improving Women's Attitudes and Coping with Menopause Symptoms. *Journal of Obstetric, Gynecologic and Neonatal Nursing* 2005; 34(2):233-240.

5. Pearson JA, Burkhart E, Pifalo WB, Palaggo-Toy T, Krohn K. A lifestyle modification intervention for the treatment of osteoporosis. *American Journal of Health Promotion* 2005; 20(1):28-33.

6. Dr Mark Porter. Decision-making with your doctor. *The Menopause Exchange Newsletter* Autumn 2003.

7. The North American Menopause Society. NAMS HRT Position Statement. *Menopause* 2008; 15(4):592.

8. Hormone Replacement Therapy: Updated Advice. Drug Safety Update. MHRA and CHM. 2007 September; 1(2).

9. Coon JT, Pittler MH, Ernst E. Trifolium pratense isoflavones in the treatment of menopausal hot flushes: A systemic review and meta-analysis. *Phytomedicine* 2007; 14:153-159.

10. Van der Sluijs CP, Bensoussan A, Liyanage L, Shah S. Women's health during mid-life survey: the use of complementary and alternative medicine by symptomatic women transitioning through menopause in Sydney. *Menopause* 2007; 14(3 Part 1):397-403.

11. Carroll DG. Nonhormonal therapies for hot flashes in menopause. *American Family Physician* 2006; 73(3):457-464.

12. Haimov-Kochman R., Hochner-Celnikier D. Hot flashes revisited: pharmacological and herbal options for hot flashes management. What does the evidence tell us? *Acta Obstetrica Gynecologica Scandinavica* 2005; 84(10):972-979.

13. National Osteoporosis Society. *Diet & Bone Health* 2006; 18.

14. Ried K, Frank OR, Stocks NP, Fakler P, Sullivan T. Effect of garlic on blood pressure: a systematic review and meta-analysis. *BMC Cardiovascular Disorders* 2008; 8(13): Review.

15. Powolny AA, Singh SV. Multi-targeted prevention and therapy of cancer by diallyl trisulfide and related allium vegetable-derived organosulfur compounds. *Cancer Letters* 2008; Jun 23.

16. UK Committee on Toxicity of Chemicals in Food, Consumer Products and the Environment, Phytoestrogens and Health 2003; Chapter 6:43 Food Standards Agency.

17. Nielsen FH, Milne DB, Klevay LM, Gallagher S, Johnson L. Dietary magnesium deficiency induces heart rhythm changes, impairs glucose tolerance, and decreases serum cholesterol in post menopausal women. *Journal of American College of Nutritionists* 2007; 26(2):21-132.

18. Howes MD. Antioxidant vitamins A, C & E; death in small doses and legal liability? 2007; PHILICA.COM. Article number 89.

19. Henderson L, Gregory J, Irving K. The National Diet and Nutrition Survey: Adults Aged 19–64 Years. 2003; (3) HMSO, London.

20. Umland EM. Treatment strategies for reducing the burden of menopause-associated vasomotor symptoms. *Journal of Managed Care Pharmacy* 2008; 14(3):14-19.

21. Kam IW, Dennehy CE, Tsourounis C. Dietary supplement use among menopausal women attending a San Francisco health conference. *Menopause* 2002; 9(1):72-78.

22. Kotsopoulos D, Dalais FS, Liang YL, McGrath BP, Teede HJ. The effects of soy protein containing phytoestrogens on menopausal symptoms in postmenopausal women. *Climacteric* 2000; 3(3):161-167.

Contact details of organisations

Bladder & Bowel Foundation
SATRA Innovation Park
Rockingham Road
Kettering
Northants NN16 9JH, UK
Tel: 01536 533255
Fax: 0870 770 3249
mailto:info@bladderandbowelfoundation.org
Web: www.bladderandbowelfoundation.org

British Association for Counselling and Psychotherapy
BACP House
15 St John's Business Park
Lutterworth
Leicestershire LE17 4HB, UK
Tel: 01455 883300
Email: bacp@bacp.co.uk
Web: www.bacp.co.uk

The British Psychological Society
St Andrew's House

48 Princess Road East
Leicester LE1 7DR, UK
Tel: 0116 254 9568
Fax: 0116 227 1314
E-mail: enquiries@bps.org.uk
Web: www.bps.org.uk

British Snoring & Sleep Apnoea Association
Castle Court
41 London Road
Reigate
RH2 9RJ, UK
Tel: 01737 245638
Fax: 0870 052 9212
E-mail: info@britishsnoring.co.uk
Web: www.britishsnoring.co.uk

The Daisy Network
The Daisy Network
PO Box 183
Rossendale
BB4 6WZ, UK
Email: daisy@daisynetwork.org.uk

Endometriosis UK
50 Westminster Palace Gardens
Artillery Row
London SW1P 1RR, UK
Tel: 020 7222 2781
Helpline: 0808 808 2227
Fax: 020 7222 2786
Email: enquiries@endometriosis-uk.org
Web: www.endometriosis-uk.org

The Hysterectomy Association

Prospect House
Peverell Avenue East
Dorchester
Dorset DT1 3WE, UK
Helpline: 0871 7811141
Fax: 01305 260676
Email: info@hysterectomy-association.org.uk
Web: www.hysterectomy-association.org.uk

The International Register of Consultant Herbalists & Homeopaths

32 King Edward Road
Swansea
West Glamorgan
SA1 4LL, UK
Tel: 01792 655886
Fax: 01792 655886
Web: www.irch.org

The Menopause Exchange

PO Box 205
Bushey
Hertfordshire WD23 1ZS, UK
Tel: 020 8420 7245
Fax: 020 8954 2783
Email: norma@menopause-exchange.co.uk
Web: www.menopause-exchange.co.uk

The National Institute of Medical Herbalists

Elm House
54 Mary Arches Street
Exeter EX4 3BA, UK

Tel: 01392 426022
Fax: 01392 498963
E-mail: info@nimh.org.uk
Web: www.nimh.org.uk

National Osteoporosis Society
Camerton
Bath
BA2 0PJ, UK
Tel: 01761 471771 / 0845 130 3076
Helpline: 0845 450 0230
Email: info@nos.org.uk
Web: www.nos.org.uk

UK Council for Psychotherapy
2nd Floor
Edward House
2 Wakley Street
London EC1V 7LT, UK
Tel: 020 7014 9955
Fax: 020 7014 9977
Email: info@psychotherapy.org.uk
Web: www.psychotherapy.org.uk

International Osteoporosis Foundation
9, rue Juste-Olivier
CH-1260 Nyon
Switzerland
Tel. +41 22 994 0100
Fax +41 22 994 0101

Index

acupressure, 70
acupuncture, 32, 70, 72, 107
agnus castus
  and mood swings, 71, 107
alcohol
  and hot flushes, 14, 80, 82-3, 105,
    106-8, 110, 122
  and HRT, 48
  and osteoporosis, risk factors for, 39,
    40, 42, 82-3, 91
  and palpitations, 13
  and sleep apnoea, 130
  and symptoms of menopause, 31
Alexander technique, 30
antidepressants, 108
  and short-term benefit, 102
  and side effects, 102
  SNRIs, 102-3, 107, 108
  SSRIs, 108
  venlafaxine (antidepressant), 102
    and hot flushes, 18,102-3, 107, 108
    improvement of libido, 102
    improvement of mood, 102
antioxidants
  and bone health, 94
  and cancer, 86, 95
  garlic, 84
  and heart disease, 95
  and menopause, 95-6
  minerals, 95
  selenium, 94
  sources of, 95
  supplements, 95

vitamin A, 95
vitamin C, 95
vitamin E, 95
anxiety, 74, 83, 101, 119
  and relaxation techniques, 119
aromatherapy, 30, 70, 72, 119
arthritis, 9, 16-18, 65-6
Asian women
  and cultural values, 8
  leaflets on menopause, 8
  onset of menopause, 8
asthma
  and HRT, 133
  and menopause, 132-3

black cohosh, 70-2
  and blood pressure medications, 71,
    113
  and breast cancer, 121
  contraindications, 71, 113
  effectiveness, 71
  and hot flushes, 71, 72, 74, 106,
    107,109
  interaction with prescription
    medicines, 74
  and libido, 115
    and liver damage, 71
  and menopausal symptoms, 71, 72
  and mood swings, 115
  and short term use, 71, 72
  and vaginal dryness, 115
bladder changes, 18-22
  and cystitis, 18-19

and incontinence pads, 21
and information on, 21
and leakage, 18-19
and medication, 18, 21
and pelvic floor exercises, 18, 20
and surgery, 18
and TENA products, 21
and urinary tract infections (UTIs),
    20, 21
and urogynaecology clinics, 21
bloating, 35, 36, 62
blood pressure
  and garlic, 4
  lowering of, 84
  testing, 128
bone-density measurement, 7, 38,
117

calcium, 91-3, 94, 98
  absorption of, 79
  bone health, maintenance of, 79,
    91, 92, 94, 105, 119
  sources, 91
  and vitamin D, 79, 92, 93
camomile tea
  as general relaxant, 74
cancer
  and antioxidants, 86
  breast, 103, 120-3
  and HRT, 135-8
    annual assessment, 138
    and black cohosh, 70-2
    and mammograms, 135
    and menopausal symptoms,
      treatment of, 120-3
    and self-examination, 135-6
    Women's Health Initiative Study
      (WHI), 137
  endometrial, 136
  and garlic, 84
carpal tunnel syndrome
  and HRT, 131
  and menopause, 131
  and treatment, 131-2
chaste tea
  and hormone imbalance, 74
cholesterol
  effect of wild yam on, 74

and garlic, 4
and impact of oestrogen and
    progesterone on, 56
lowering levels of, 81-2, 84,96
and oestrogen implants, 53
testing, 104, 112, 128
clonidine
  and high blood pressure, 102, 103
  and menopausal symptoms, 73,
    102, 103, 108
  and migraine, 102
  and side effects, 102, 103
concentration, poor, 10
copper, 95

Daisy Network, Premature
    Menopause Support Group, 6
depression, 28, 66-7, 83
dietary supplements, 78, 82, 84-100
  antioxidants, 84, 89, 90, 94-7
  advice, importance of professional,
    78, 89-90
  calcium, 91-2, 94
  fish oils, 89, 97-9
  garlic, 84-5, 89
  interaction with prescribed
    medication, 78
  iron, 95
  magnesium, 93-4
  selenium, 94
  and vaginal dryness, 115-16
  vitamin D, 90, 94
  see also phytoestrogens, soya
digestive problems. 9, 35
dizziness, 10
Dong quai
  and contraindications, 75
  effectiveness, 75
  and hot flushes, 74

early onset of menopause, 7
  and age, 5
  and hysterectomy, 3
  and smoking, 118-19
emotional symptoms, 28-34
  anxiety, 29
  and counselling, 29, 30
  depression, 28-9

post-hysterectomy, 28
and exercise, 28, 32
mood swings, 29-30
and natural remedies, 28
panic attacks, 30
stress, 33
and stress management, 28, 30,
    33-4
and support groups, 29
endometriosis
Endometriosis UK, 126
and treatment,126
evening primrose oil
and dry skin, 23-4
and hot flushes. 76
exercise
and anxiety, 119
and bladder leakage, 18-19
and bloating, 36
and depression, 28
and dry mouth, 27
and emotional problems, 32
and fatigue, 64, 114
and hair loss, 26, 99
and health checks for HRT, 48
and hot flushes, 106, 107
and irritability, 31
and joint stiffness, 17
and libido, 117
and menopausal symptoms, 101, 118
and mood swings, 119
and nails, 99
and night sweats, 107
and osteoarthritis, 17
and osteoporosis, 39-40, 91, 119
and stress, 33
and vaginal dryness, 21
and weight problems, 34-5, 62, 106
exhaustion, 77
expectations of menopause, 3
  and biological factors, 16
  cultural beliefs, 3, 16
  and depression, 3, 16
  onset, suddenness of, 3
eye problems, 12, 60

facial hair, 25-6
false unicorn root,

and hormone imbalance, 74
fatigue, 33
and exercise, 64, 114
Ferrum metallicum
and exhaustion, 77
and hot flushes, 77
fibroids
and HRT, 124
and menopause, 124-5
myomectomy, 125
and treatment, 125
fluoxetine
and hot flushes, 122
flushes, hot, 2, 3, 4, 7, 9, 12
and agnus castus, 71, 107
and alcohol, 14, 80, 82-3, 105,
    106-8, 110, 122
and black cohosh, 71, 72, 74, 106,
    107, 109
and caffeine, 80
and clonidine, 73, 102, 103,
    108,121
and Dong quai, 74
and evening primrose oil, 76
and exercise, 106, 107
and gabapentin, 102, 111, 121
and 'hyperventilation', 14
and increased stress, 33
isoflavones (phytoestrogens), 79,
    107, 109
lignans (phytoestrogens), 79
and nutrition, 79-80
and phytoestrogens 71, 74, 78, 80,
    109, 111
and progestogens, 108, 121
and red clover, 71
and spicy foods, 80
St John's Wort, 74
and venlafaxine (antidepressant),
    18,102-3, 107, 111
and vitamin E, 99

gabapentin
and hot flushes, 111
and side effects, 111
garlic
and anti-clotting properties, 84
antioxidant, 84

and blood pressure lowering effect, 84-5
and cholesterol-lowering effect, 4, 84-5
gum problems, 26-7

hair problems, 9, 25-6, 56-8, 99, 114-15
headaches, 11-12
heart disease
and exercise 80
and garlic, 84
and nutrition, 79
and phytoestrogens, 85
and selenium, 94
herbal remedies, 54, 55, 71-5, 111
advice, importance of professional, 70-1, 73, 74, 77, 109, 110
agnus castus, 71, 107
black cohosh, 70, 71-3, 74, 106, 107, 109, 113, 115, 121
chaste tea, 74
clinical trials, lack of, 72, 73, 75, 76
interaction with prescribed medications, 71, 73, 74, 110
contraindications, 71, 72, 74, 109
effectiveness of, 71
false unicorn root, 74
isoflavones (phytoestrogens), 72, 109
Menoherbs 2, 110
phytoestrogens
and hot flushes, 74, 109, 111
and long term safety, 74
red clover, 71, 107, 113, 115
sage, 113
short term use, 74
and vaginal symptoms, 115-16
wild yam, 74
valerian, 129
homeopathy, 70, 71
Ferrum metallicum, 77
and hot flushes, 77, 106
Lachesis mutus, 77
Lycopodium clavatum, 77
and mood swings, 77
Pulsatilla, 77
Sepia, 77
Sulphur, 77

Valerian, 77
hormone replacement therapy, see HRT
hospital menopause service, 8
HRT (hormone replacement therapy), 10, 43-69
and age spots, 25
and alcohol, 48
and arthritis, 65-6
and asthma, 132-3
and bleeding, 43, 46-7
and bloating, 62
and blood pressure, 60
and breast cancer, 21, 63, 121-3, 138
and risk of, 135-8
and bypassing symptoms, 59-60
and carpal tunnel syndrome, 131
and contact lenses, 60
and contraception, 50-2, 61
contraindications, 44-5
continuous combined, 43, 47, 62
and deep vein thrombosis (DVT), 61, 64, 138
and depression, 66-7
and diabetes, 55-6
and early menopause, 68-9
effectiveness of, 54
and endometrial cancer, 43
and fertility, 50-2
and fibroids, 123
and formication (itchy skin), 22, 23
and hair problems, 56-7
and health checks, 48-9
and hot flushes, 12,16, 43, 49, 54, 55, 63, 107-8, 11, 122
and hysterectomy, 43, 46, 63, 64, 66
and improvement in symptoms, 49
intrauterine system (IUS), 44, 47-8
and joint stiffness, 17
long-cycle, 43
and libido, loss of, 52, 54, 55, 116-17
and long haul flights, 61
and memory, 121
and migraines, 63
and Mirena coil, 47
and mood swings, 43

and natural ingredients, 45-6
and night sweats, 43
oestrogen implants, 52-4
oestrogen-only, 43, 44, 53-54, 63,
    136
oestrogen and progesterone
    combined, 43, 46, 56, 63, 137
    forms of, 44
    types of, 43
and osteoporosis, 65, 66, 67-8
and palpitations, 12
patches, 45, 50, 58, 62;
    removal of marks, 55
and patient choice, 18, 44
and phytoestrogens, 88
and premature menopause, 5, 10
prescription charges, 48
    protection for bones, 12
and pulmonary embolism (PE), 61, 64
and reduction, gradual, 17, 58-9,
    106-7, 111
risk-benefit evaluation, 68, 76, 107
risks, 8, 21, 68
sequential combined (cyclical
    combined), 43, 47, 62
and sex life, 52
side effects, 8, 25, 54
and skin dryness, 25
and skin pigmentation, changes in,
    22
and sleep disturbance, 128-9
and spine and hip fractures, 43
and stroke, 138
and surgery, 58-9
tablets, 58, 62
and testosterone, 55, 66
and treatment of menopause, 8,
    43-69
and urinary problems, 43
and vaginal dryness, 22, 43, 49, 54
and varicose veins, 61
and weight gain, 62
hypnotherapy, 70
hysterectomy
and early onset of menopause, 3
and exercise, 123
and fibroids, 125
and healthy diet, 123

and HRT, 43, 54, 66, 136
Hysterectomy Association, The,
    123, 146

Implants
    advantages, 52-3
    disadvantages, 52-4
    insertion of, 52-33
    and oestrogen only HRT, 52-3
    and tachyphylaxis, 53-4
intrauterine system (IUS),
    Mirena coil, 47-8
    and progesterone part of HRT,
        44, 47-8
iron, 79, 90
    sources of, 95
irritability, 30-1
isoflavones (phytoestrogens)
    and menopausal symptoms, 72-3,
        107, 108, 117
    sage 73
    soya, 73, 117

joint problems, 9,16-18
    and exercise, 17
    and glucosamine, 17

Lachesis Mutus
    and hot flushes, 77
libido, loss of, 52, 54, 74
    and counselling, 116
    and exercise, 117
    and HRT, 116, 117
    and medication side effects, 116
    and prescription medicines, 117
    and stress, 116
    and testosterone implant, 117
    and vaginal dryness, 116
lignans (phytoestrogens)
    and menopausal symptoms, 79
    fibre-rich foods, 79
lime blossom tea
    as general relaxant, 74
Lycopodium clavatum
    and vaginal dryness, 77

magnesium, 79, 93
    and bone health, 94

manganese, 95
ME (myalgic encephalomyelitis)
 symptoms, 132
meditation, 70, 119
memory loss, 10, 121
menopause clinics, 6-7, 55, 115
 referral to other services, 7
menopause, options for coping with,
 101-19
menopausal status
 follicle stimulating hormone (FSH),
 50-1
Menopause Exchange, The, vii, xi,
 xiii, 120, 146
migraines, 11, 62-3, 111
minerals, 78, 95, 99
 and age, 90
 and bone protection, 93-4
 calcium, 91-3, 94, 94, 98
 copper, 95
 interaction with supplements and
 prescription medicine, 89
 iron, 79, 95
 magnesium, 79,93
 manganese, 95
 selenium, 79, 94, 95
 zinc, 95
mood swings, 10, 71,77, 80, 105-6,
 107, 108, 115
 and exercise, 80, 119
 and relaxation techniques, 119
mouth problems, 9, 26-7

National Osteoporosis Society, 91
nutrition 78-100
 and cancer, 79
 general, 78, 79-84
 and heart disease, 79, 80
 and hot flushes, 79, 80, 101
 and joints, 79
 vitamin D, 79
 and menopause, 79-80
 phytoestrogens, 84-8
 prebiotics, 82
 probiotics, 82
 and saturated fats, 79, 81
 vitamins and minerals, 88-100
 and weight gain, 79, 80

oats
 as gentle tonic, 74
oestrogen implants, 52-4
 advantages, 53
 and cholesterol, 53
 disadvantages, 53
 dosage, 53
 insertion of, 53
 and tachyphylaxis, 53-4
onset of menopause, 1
 age, average, 4, 5, 10, 13, 14, 39,
 49, 54, 66, 69, 125
 and Asian women, 8
 and blood test, 4, 6, 51
 and cancer, 5
 and contraception, 50-2
 diagnosis, 38
 early, 3, 5, 7
 and expectations, 3
 and fertility, 50-2
 and follicle stimulating hormone
 (FSH), 51-2
 and hysterectomy, 3
 ovaries, surgical removal of, 5
 premature, 5, 6, 10
osteoarthritis
 and exercise, 17
osteoporosis, 12, 37-42
 and alcohol, 39, 40, 42, 82-3, 91
 and bisphosphonates, 68
 and calcium intake, 42
 diagnosis, 38
 and exercise, 39-41, 91, 119
 and general nutrition, 79-84
 and HRT, 67-8;
 and immobility, 64
 and natural progesterone cream, 75
 and oestrogen, lack of, 38
 and phytoestrogens, 84-8
 prevention of, 40-1
 risk factors, 39-40, 104
 and smoking, 119
 and vitamins and minerals, 89-100;
 see also individual vitamins and
 minerals
 and weight-bearing exercise, 40-2,
 80

palpitations
  and alcohol, 13
  and caffeine, 12, 13
  and stress, 13
  and tiredness, 13
passiflora tablets
  and tension and anxiety, 74
perimenopause, 35
  and dry skin, 24
  and headaches, 11
period pains, 130-1
phytoestrogens
  and breast cancer, 86
  and contraindications, 85-6
  and dose, 87
  and heart disease, 85
  and hot flushes, 71, 74, 122
  and HRT, 88
  and interaction with prescribed
    medication, 85-6
  isoflavones, 72, 79, 86
  lignans, 79
  red clover, 71, 107
  sage, 73, 113
  and short term use, 72, 74, 111
  and side effects, 85
  soya, 85, 88-8, 111
  as supplements, 87-8
  and thyroxine, 85-6
post-natal depression, 2
premature menopause, 5, 6
  and cyopreservation of ovarian
    tissue, 6
  familial tendency, 6
  and fertility, 6
  and HRT, 5, 10
  prevention of, 6
premenstrual syndrome, 3
  and Dong quai, 75
    and menopausal symptoms, 101
progestogens
  and breast cancer, 76
  and endometrial cancer, 136
  and hot flushes, 108
  and menopausal symptoms, 75
  and osteoporosis, 75
Pulsatilla
  as homeopathic remedy, 77

red clover
  and hot flushes, 71, 72, 107, 113
relaxation techniques, 32
  acupuncture, 31
  Alexander technique, 31
  aromatherapy, 31, 119
  yoga, 32, 119
reflexology, 70, 72
relaxation, 70
rheumatoid arthritis
  and omega-3 oils, 98-9

sage
  and blood pressure medication, 113
  and breast cancer, 73
  and hormonal imbalance, 74
  and hot flushes, 73
  interaction with prescribed
    medications, 73
  isoflavones (phytoestrogens), 73
  and sore throats, 73
  and sweating, 73, 74
selenium, 79, 95
  and antioxidant effects, 94
  and heart disease, 94
  sources of, 94
Sepia
  as homeopathic remedy, 77
skin problems, 9, 22-5, 114-15
  and HRT, 25
  and oestrogen cream, 24
  and moisturisers and emollients,
    24, 25
  and pessaries, 24
sleep apnoea, 130
  and alcohol, 130
snoring, 129-30
SNRIs (antidepressants)
  and hot flushes, 102-3, 107, 108
  Venlafaxine, 102
SSRIs (antidepressants),
  and hot flushes, 108
soya
  and bones, 42
  health risks, 88-9
  and hot flushes, 85, 105, 111,113,
    116, 117
  isoflavones (phytoestrogens), 117

and libido, 115
and mood swings, 115
as supplement, 87-9
and thyroxine, 85-6
and vaginal dryness, 115
St John's Wort
 and anxiety, 119
 and hot flushes, 74
 and mood swings, 119
stages of menopause,
 menopause itself, 2
 perimenopause, 2, 10, 14, 24, 35,
  105
  and contraception, 104
  and HRT, 4
  and smoking, 119
 post-menopause, 2, 12, 19,115-16,
  127
  and bloating, 35
  and HRT, 47
stress, 14, 16, 27, 33, 99
Sulphur
 and night sweats, 77
support groups, 29
sweats, night, 2, 7, 8, 9, 10, 13-16,
  34, 51, 64, 77, 101, 103, 106, 110
symptoms, 1, 2, 3, 9-36
 and acne, 133-4
 and acupuncture, 32, 70, 72,
  107,123
 and agnus castus, 71, 107
 and alcohol,14, 31, 80, 82-3, 105,
  106, 107, 110,122
 and allergies, 133
 and alternative medicines, 18
 and alternative remedies, 31
 and antidepressants, 102
 anxiety, 74, 83, 101, 119
 arthritis, 9, 16-18, 65-6
 and black cohosh, 71-3, 106, 107
 bladder changes, 9, 10, 18-22
 bloating, 35, 62
 and caffeine, 12, 13, 14, 30, 33, 36,
  83, 106, 107, 110
 and camomile tea, 74
 carpal tunnel syndrome, 131
 and changes in temperature, 14
 and chaste tea, 74

and cigarettes, 33
and clonidine, 73, 102, 103, 108
and clothing, 14, 16
concentration, poor, 10
depression, 66-7, 83
and diet, 30, 31, 33, 34, 36, 80, 104,
  105, 114, 119; see also dietary
  supplements, nutrition
dietary supplements, 18
digestive problems, 9, 35
dizziness, 10
emotional, 9, 10, 28-34
and evening primrose oil, 76
and eyes
 dry eyes, 60
 eyesight, 12, 60
and exercise, 30, 31, 32, 33, 34, 36,
  99, 101, 104, 114, 118, 119
exhaustion, 77
facial hair, 25-6
and false unicorn root, 74
fatigue 33
and fluid intake, 14, 16
flushes, hot, 2, 3, 4, 7, 9, 10, 12,13-
  16, 34, 39, 51, 54, 55, 63-4, 76,
  77, 101, 102-3, 105-13, 115, 117
 and black cohosh, 71, 72, 74, 106,
  107, 109
 and herbal remedies, 71, 109
 and 'hyperventilation', 14
 and lifestyle changes, 101
 and nutrition, 79-80
 and self-help measures, 101
 and tingling, 14
 and vitamin E, 99
 and fluoxetine (antidepressant), 122
formication (itchy skin), 22, 23
and gabapentin, 102, 108
general, 9, 10-13
and gingko biloba, 121
gums, 26-7
hair problems, 9, 25-6, 56-8, 99,
  114-15
headaches, 11-12
and heat loss, 14
and HRT, 5, 8, 10, 12, 16, 17, 18,
  20, 21, 22, 25, 43-69; and
  bypassing symptoms, 59-60

and homeopathy, 70, 71, 77, 106
and hypnotherapy, 123
and isoflavones, 72
itchy skin (formication), 22, 23
joint problems, 9, 16-18, 111
libido, loss of, 52, 54
and lime blossom tea, 74
memory loss, 10, 121:
   and Bach flower, 121
migraines, 11, 62-3, 111
mood swings, 10,71,77, 80, 105-6,
   107, 108, 115,119
mouth problems, 9, 26-7
and natural progesterone cream, 75
and non-oestrogen-based treatment,
   102, 107, 111
onset of, 9
and oestrogen implants, 52-4
osteoporosis, 12, 37-42, 83, 104
palpitations, 12, 13, 111
and passiflora tablets, 74
and phytoestrogens, 71, 72, 73, 74,
   78-9, 84-8, 100, 107, 122
and prescription medicine, 101,
   102
and progestogens, 73, 102
and relaxation techniques, 31, 32,
   33
and sage, 73
skin problems, 9, 22-5, 114-15
and sleep disturbance, 129
and smoking, 104, 119-20
and spicy food, 14, 106
and stress, 14, 16, 27, 33, 99
sweats, night, 2, 7, 8, 9,10, 13-16,
   34, 39, 51, 64, 77, 101, 103, 106,
   110
and tamoxifen, 122
tension, 74
vaginal changes, 9, 10, 18-22, 24-5,
   54, 77, 115-16, 117, 121
and valerian, 129
vasomotor, 39, 60, 107, 108
and venlafaxine (antidepressant),
   102-3, 107, 122
and vitamins and minerals, 89-100;
   see also individual vitamins and
   minerals

weight problems, 34-5, 83, 114
and wild yam, 74

Tai chi, 32, 33, 70
tachyphylaxis
   and HRT implants, 53-4
therapies, complementary, 70-7, 101,
   107
   acupressure, 70
   acupuncture, 30, 32, 71, 72, 100
   advice, importance of, 70-1, 73,
      74, 77
   aromatherapy, 70, 72
   herbal medicine, 70, 71-5; see also
      herbal remedies
   homeopathy, 70, 71
   hypnotherapy, 70
   interaction with medication, 71
   meditation, 70
   reflexology, 70, 72, 110
   relaxation, 70
   Tai chi, 32, 33, 70
   yoga, 70, 110

uterus, double chamber, 127
   and pregnancy, 127

vaginal changes, 18-22
   atrophic vaginitis, 19, 22
   and black cohosh, 115
   and dietary supplements, 115-16
   and dryness, 19, 21, 115
   and isoflavone creams, 116
   and loss of libido, 116-17
   and oestrogen cream, 22, 54, 117,
      121
   and pessaries, 54
   and exercise, 22
   and HRT, 22
   itchy skin, 24-5
   and KY jelly, 19, 116
   and pessaries, 20, 21, 22, 24
   and red clover, 20
   and sex, 22
Valerian
   and night sweats, 77
vasomotor symptoms, 39, 60, 107,
   108; see also flushes, hot and

sweats, night
acupuncture, 107
and antidepressants, 108
and clonidine, 108
and gabapentin, 108
and herbal medicine, 107
and HRT, 107-8
and isoflavones (phytoestrogens), 107
and lifestyle changes, 107,108
and prescription progestogens, 108
venlafaxine (antidepressant)
  and breast cancer, 103
  and hot flushes, 18, 102 , 107, 111, 122
  improvement of libido, 102
  improvement of mood, 102
  and side effects, 111
vitamin supplements
 A, 79, 89
  antioxidant properties, 95
  and liver damage, 97
  sources, 96
  and osteoporosis, 98
 B group, 79, 90
  folic acid, 100

C, 79
  antioxidant properties, 95
D, 79, 89:
  and bone health, 94
  and skin cancer, 93
  and sunlight, 90, 92, 93
E, 79
  antioxidant properties, 95
  side effects, 99
  and calcium absorption, 79

weight problems, 34-5, 74, 83, 114
  and diet, 34
  and exercise, 34-5, 62, 106
  and heart disease, 34
  and high cholesterol, 81
wild yam
  and cholesterol, 74
  and hormone imbalance, 74

yoga, 32, 34, 70

zinc, 95

About the Author

Norma Goldman BPharm. MRPharmS. MSc. is the Founder and Director of The Menopause Exchange, the independent information service for women experiencing menopausal symptoms or needing help at the post-menopause, and also for health professionals. She is a pharmacist and qualified health promotion specialist, having obtained a Master's degree in health promotion in 1996. Following this she went on to found The Menopause Exchange in 1999 with the aim of providing a reliable independent source of up-to-date, impartial, practical and easily understood information on all aspects of the menopause in the form of quarterly newsletters, fact sheets and an information service. The Menopause Exchange has its own 'Ask the experts' panel to answer members' questions. Because of feedback received by members about the answers to their questions, she realised that these would be of interest and use to other women, and so decided to put them into book form, encouraged by Hammersmith Press. Because of her qualifications, knowledge and her work as a speaker on all aspects of the menopause to both women and health professionals, she is constantly researching new and up-to-date information and is highly attuned to the concerns of women facing the menopause and their families and friends.